In clear prose, Jos de Kroon presents an alternative to current psychiatry, which seems to have had its day. His point of departure is a structuralist approach in which more space and freedom are reserved for the subject.

Professor Marc De Kesel, *Radboud University, Nijmegen, the Netherlands*

A Structuralist Approach in Psychiatry is an atypical psychiatric book that challenges the dominant naturalistic and mechanistic paradigms of contemporary psychiatry. While engaging with crucial questions of diagnosis and treatment, it critiques mainstream psychiatric discourse through the lens of structuralist linguistics, Lacanian psychoanalysis, and continental philosophy. De Kroon argues for a structuralist psychiatry that recognizes the subject as fundamentally shaped by its symbolic and discursive environment, rather than reducing mental illness to neurobiological determinants. Through a nuanced reading of concepts from Saussure, Lacan, Heidegger, and Žižek, he explores how "nothingness" operates as a creative force in subject formation and in psychosis. With case discussions on Cotard's syndrome, Capgras syndrome, and negative hallucinations, the book demonstrates how symbolic disruptions manifest in clinical practice. Rather than merely confronting psychiatry with philosophy, De Kroon constructs a bridge between psychoanalytic theory and psychiatric treatment, making a compelling plea for a paradigm shift in mental health care.

Professor Stijn Vanheule, *University of Ghent, Belgium*

A STRUCTURALIST APPROACH IN PSYCHIATRY

A Structuralist Approach in Psychiatry presents an alternative view of the psychiatric patient and highlights a connection with continental post-structuralist thinking to provide a new approach to psychiatry.

After outlining the problems facing psychiatry and the historical development of the field, this book outlines a structuralist model of the subject that does greater justice to the complexity involved while avoiding physicalist reductionism. It draws heavily on French structuralism, in which language plays a central structuring role that also influences the subject. The author draws on the works of Foucault, Lacan, and Bergson, as well as Nietzsche, Heidegger, and Žižek. The structuralist model proposed engages with the intricate relationships between the Real, the Imaginary, and the Symbolic in relation to the subject, particularly in the marginality of psychosis. Three clinical examples are provided to illustrate this: the syndromes of Cotard, Capgras, and negative hallucination. These examples demonstrate how the negative within the subject manifests itself in their symptomatology. However, the negative also plays a role in the normal development of the subject when they encounter the Symbolic and enter the world of language. Time and again, the subject must reinvent themselves through speech. This model, grounded in the concept of the zero point, has implications for an alternative anthropology and for psychiatry, where speaking and listening take center stage.

This book will be of interest to mental healthcare professionals, including psychiatric nurses, psychiatrists, psychologists, and physician assistants, and those studying to enter these professions.

Jos de Kroon is a psychiatrist, psychotherapist, and psychoanalyst working at the Reinier van Arkel Institution of Mental Health in Den Bosch, the Netherlands. He publishes on the subjects of psychiatry and science, Freud, and Lacan. His publications include *Language and psychosis* (1993), *The history of psychiatry* (1999), *About the soul* (2007), *The voice of the Other* (2010, about verbal hallucinations), and *Hamlet versus Oedipus or a matrixial orientation?* (2020), and *Discomfort and Desire—A Lacanian View of the Subject in the Age of Artificial Intelligence* (2026).

A STRUCTURALIST APPROACH IN PSYCHIATRY

Uncanny and Desire in Psychosis

Jos de Kroon

Routledge
Taylor & Francis Group
NEW YORK AND LONDON

Designed cover image: © Giorgio de Chirico, La Maschere 1, 1918 c/o Pictoright Amsterdam 2025

First published in English 2026
by Routledge
605 Third Avenue, New York, NY 10158

and by Routledge
4 Park Square, Milton Park, Abingdon, Oxon, OX14 4RN

Routledge is an imprint of the Taylor & Francis Group, an informa business

Published in Dutch by Garant Publishers 2021

ISBN: 978-1-041-14632-2 (hbk)
ISBN: 978-1-041-03105-5 (pbk)
ISBN: 978-1-003-67538-9 (ebk)

DOI: 10.4324/9781003675389

Typeset in Sabon
by SPi Technologies India Pvt Ltd (Straive)

For Olga Viltovskaya

CONTENTS

Acknowledgments *xii*
Preface *xiv*

Introduction 1

PART 1
Positioning of Modern Psychiatry **5**

1 Outline of the Problem Facing Psychiatry 11

2 Historical Development of Psychiatry from the Enlightenment 16

PART 2
Structuralism and Nothingness **23**

3 Structuralism 27

4 Fundamental Impossibilities 32

5 Nothingness and Science 36

6 Nothingness as a Creative Moment 39

PART 3
Three Experiences of Nothingness in the Clinic **43**

7 As in a Black Mirror: Cotard's Syndrome 47

8 The Stranger in Ourselves: Capgras Syndrome 58

9 The Experience of Nothingness 64

PART 4
Towards a Different Perspective of the Subject **75**

10 Subject and Science 79

11 Looking for the Psyche in Psychiatry 90

12 Sketch of an Alternative 94

PART 5
The Creative Power of Nothingness **101**

13 Friedrich Nietzsche and Degree Zero of Morality 103

14 Interlude: Fable 106

15 Martin Heidegger and Nothingness 108

16 Nothingness at Jacques Lacan 117

17 Slavoj Žižek: Can It Be Less Than Nothing? 121

18 Genealogy of Creation 128

19 Toward a Structuralist Psychiatry 132

20 The Role of Linguistics in a Therapeutic Perspective 137

21 The Eclipse of the (Psychotic) Subject? 141

22 What About the Self? 150

PART 6
To Resist the Death Instinct of Nothingness: An Investigation into Nothingness as the Ground of Desire **157**

23 An Object Relations Theory Without an Object 159

24 Psychiatry and the Transcendental 166

25 The Ethical Implications of Mysticism and Desire 170

26 The Subject as a Dynamic Process: From Deadlock to Transformation-Symbolization as a Response to Nothingness 174

27 Everything or Nothing: *About Mysticism and the Genesis of the Subject* 178

Bibliography *184*
Index of names *193*
Index of subjects *195*

ACKNOWLEDGMENTS

This book was written during my work in the clinic, in outpatient care, as well as in private praxis, where I mainly had contact with patients experiencing psychotic vulnerability. Through continuous dialogue with them, I gained some understanding of their world.

I also owe much to my colleagues, particularly mental health workers, psychoanalysts among them, and the residents training to become psychiatrists. Through constant exchange and dialogue with them, I was able to further develop my vision of psychotic disorders and the ways in which therapeutic engagement can transform clinical practice. Their collaboration has been instrumental, and I am profoundly thankful for the shared intellectual and clinical journey.

To ensure linguistic clarity and align this text with the conventions of the Anglo-Saxon discourse in mental health care, I was fortunate to have the assistance of Alf Gillham. His meticulous review of the manuscript not only helped correct errors but also enhanced the readability and precision of the work. I am grateful for his commitment and expertise.

Beyond psychiatry, I greatly benefited from my interactions with Marc De Kesel, who repeatedly guided me through the ideas of Freud and Lacan.

Toward the end of completing this book, I had the privilege of hearing Jaakko Seikkula speak at the ISPS Congress in Perugia. His lecture on Mikhail Bakhtin and his relation to Open Dialogue resonated deeply with me. I was struck by the parallels between my Lacan-inspired views and the open dialogue practices developed by Seikkula. This realization remains a path yet to be fully explored, and I am grateful to him for this inspiration.

This book represents not only a personal journey but also a collaborative endeavor shaped by the voices of patients, colleagues, and thinkers who have accompanied me along the way. To all of them, I extend my deepest gratitude.

Finally, I would like to express my gratitude to my wife, Olga Viltovskaya, for her natural generosity in allowing me the time to write this book.

PREFACE

Any psychiatrist—as well as anyone working in the field of mental health care—knows how it feels when, at certain moments in his professional career, the body of knowledge he has at his disposal reaches its limits when facing the specific tangle of psychic problems his particular patient is in. It is not to say that his knowledge suddenly appears to be entirely useless, but the singularity of his patient's problems compels the mental care professional to reflect upon, to readjust, or even to substantially revise his theoretical know-how. Practice is not simply the place where theory is applied; it is also the origin from which every genuine theory starts. At the end of the day, every reliable theory about mental health care starts from the mental health care practice.

The theoretical book Dr. Jos de Kroon presents us here reveals at every page that it has its origin in the practice of his career as a psychiatrist. This is one of the reasons for his structuralist approach. For what is the core of his structuralism's intuition? That the health care provider is not able to approach his patient and his problems as simply the object of neutral observation to whom he can apply his scientific knowledge. Therefore, the psychiatrist is too much involved in the process of giving care itself. Irrespective of his own intentions, he immediately becomes part of the patient's problematic relation to the world and to himself. Inevitably, the psychiatrist is always already himself an "object" in the field of problems his patient is in, and to that position the psychiatrist has no "objective" access. This is why a structuralist approach is needed here, an approach taking for granted the "structural" place both the psychiatrist and the patient are in.

This necessitates the psychiatrist to review the classical notion of "subject." As a psychiatrist, he is no longer a kind of "Cartesian" subject having self-assured mastery over his relation to an object, i.e., his patient. The psychiatrist is "subject"—in the sense of "subjected"—to a relation to his patient, and that position cannot be considered as based in self-assured mastery neither over itself nor the self of his patient.

It is the merit of De Kroon's approach that he puts that insight in the broader scope not only of the scientific literature of psychiatric studies but of the literature in the field of critical philosophy as well. Of that openness testifies De Kroon's use of the theory of the subject by Jacques Lacan as well. Putting that theory in a clarifying dialogue with other theoretical narratives involved in psychiatric theory and practice is not the least of the credits of this book.

Marc De Kesel, April 13, 2025

INTRODUCTION

This book presents an alternative perspective on psychiatric patients by incorporating insights from continental (post)structuralist thinkers such as Roland Barthes, Michel Foucault, Jacques Lacan, and Slavoj Žižek. Its focus is on the *subject*—as opposed to the *object*—a dimension that is often underemphasized in contemporary medicine, particularly in psychiatry. The subject emerges from a state of zero, develops within familial and societal contexts, and may either evolve into a life of richness and creativity or devolve into psychotic constellations. This framework challenges the dominant monolithic naturalistic discourse in psychiatry, advocating instead for a model aligned with Engel's biopsychosocial approach.

Relation to Other Literature

The literature referenced in this book primarily originates from fields outside traditional medicine and psychiatry. By weaving these perspectives into the discussion of psychosis, the book offers a distinctive contribution to psychiatric discourse. Conceptual parallels are drawn with methodologies such as Lacanian discourse, Gregory Bateson's Ecology of mind, and Jaakko Seikkula's Open Dialogue, highlighting shared touchpoints.

Intended Audience

This book is aimed at mental health professionals seeking a nuanced understanding of the complex "patient-subject." It is particularly relevant

DOI: 10.4324/9781003675389-1

to psychiatric nurses, psychologists, physicians, nurse specialists, psychiatrists, and trainees in psychiatry.

A Plea for Structuralist Psychiatry

This book is a heartfelt plea for a structuralist approach to psychiatry—one that does greater justice to the complexity of psychopathology than the prevailing mechanistic paradigm. Structuralist psychiatry acknowledges the profound influence of the environment on the formation of the subject. From birth, individuals are shaped by the structures and events of their surroundings, which may foster either harmonious development or pathological patterns. Essentially, the subject is structured by what happens to them.

The structuralist perspective explored in this book originates in the French-speaking intellectual tradition, profoundly influenced by the groundbreaking linguistics of Ferdinand de Saussure, as articulated in his seminal *Cours de linguistique générale* (1916). This linguistic foundation inspired a lineage of thinkers, including Claude Lévi-Strauss, Michel Foucault, Jacques Derrida, and Jacques Lacan. Their work serves as a conceptual backbone for this text, referenced where relevant. Particular attention is devoted to the role of environmental factors in structuring the subject, with a specific focus on the Lacanian concept of the relationship with the *Other* as central to this process.

While this structuring often unfolds smoothly, disruptions or deviations—what Lacan might call *fause routes*—can occur, giving rise to the psychopathological phenomena explored in this book. At the heart of the interaction between subject and Other lies a fundamental law Lacan terms the *Name-of-the-Father*. When this law is disregarded or rejected, the consequences for the subject can be profound, manifesting in conditions such as personality disorders and psychosis.

A recurring theme is that the subject must invent itself—often starting from a "zero position"—by drawing upon external materials. This paradoxical interplay between the internal and external, a concept Lacan terms *extimacy*, will be examined and elaborated throughout the text.

Reflecting on a Career in Psychiatry

After 45 years in the field of psychiatry, it feels timely to take stock of my experiences and reflections. At the time of writing, I am still actively working in a crisis service focused on preventing inpatient admissions. While we often succeed, there are occasions when we do not. The introduction of new mental health legislation in the Netherlands on January 1, 2020, aimed to reduce hospitalizations and improve patients' legal protections. However, the outcomes remain uncertain. My impression is that forced admissions and coercive measures have increased, diverging from the intended spirit of the law. Meanwhile, mental health professionals face a growing burden of administrative tasks, detracting from what I believe remains the essence of effective psychiatric care: listening to and talking with patients.

Amid this increasing mechanization of psychiatry—a central critique of this book—there remains a glimmer of hope. I see countless mental health professionals working with immense dedication and compassion, often guided by intuition rather than rigid protocols and guidelines. Despite the system's challenges, they strive tirelessly to improve their patients' lives. My admiration for these colleagues is profound.

A Vision for Psychiatry

This book offers a critique of modern psychiatry and challenges prevailing norms and assumptions. I am aware that it may provoke discomfort by confronting ideas and developments I strongly oppose. Yet my aim is not merely to critique but also to propose a conceptual model that fosters greater freedom and creativity for both patients and mental health professionals. This model seeks to integrate psychological and physical dimensions with cultural and social contexts, presenting psychiatry as a more holistic and humane discipline.

It is a challenging subject, and I make no apologies for strong statements that may touch on sensitive issues. Ultimately, however, it is up to you, the reader, to decide whether I have succeeded in this endeavor.

PART 1

Positioning of Modern Psychiatry

Introduction

After a critique of the naturalistic approach that dominates contemporary psychiatry and which is supported by a materialistic view of man through mainly Anglo-Saxon philosophy, an alternative is put forward. The subject's birth begins with nothingness, a consequence of the separation between mother and child. With this gap that has arisen, a desire to fill this void arises. When something goes wrong in this process, we see it in the psychopathology of which clinical examples are given: the syndromes of Cotard and Capgras and the phenomenon of negative hallucination. A short sketch of the history of the view of man, leading to an indication of a critical attitude towards a materialistic and controlling attitude towards psychiatric patients, closes this part.

In recent decades, academic psychiatry in particular has shown a strong preference for a naturalistic approach, which has greatly affected the attention for psychological aspects. I have always preferred to seek a balance between the somatic and the psychological in psychiatry. That balance between both orientations is now hard to find. Not only does academic psychology seek its salvation in the functioning of the brain, but also some psychoanalysts seek their basis in neuropsychoanalysis (cf. Mark Solms). It seems that the psychological in man no longer has a say because it is not accessible to science that focuses on the observable and the measurable. The psychological is placed by science under the metaphysical and the transcendental, which is not measurable and objectifiable. That is correct because it belongs to the subjective, which is essentially of a different order

DOI: 10.4324/9781003675389-2

than the objective. In psychiatry, and especially where psychopathology is concerned, we will have to focus on a two-track policy and accept the insoluble nature of the soma-psycho problem and not think that reduction of the psychic into the somatic is a solution to the problem.

This text aims to be an outline of an alternative to a far-reaching materialisation of psychiatry. In psychiatric circles, it is common practice to project everything that is human into the workings of the brain and to pour a scientific sauce over it, a sauce that initially pleases us but does violence to the psychological reality. If a product, a government decision, or a method is to be successful with the public, they must bear the scientific designation. It is no different in psychiatry. Psychotropic drugs and treatment methods must be scientifically proven to have any authority. The psychiatric literature is inundated with Randomised Controlled Trials (RCTs) to ensure its truth. The overwhelming amount of data that this yielded has not brought psychiatry much further since 1953, when the first psychotropic drugs came on the market. Imaging techniques such as the CT scan and fMRI are highly regarded for their ability to visualise the damaged and functioning brain, which has fuelled the idea for some that the mind-body problem has been solved because it has now become clear that all psychological functions are brain functions. The opposite is true. The background to this mistake is widely discussed in this book. In the meantime, materialistic thinking is expanding in psychiatry and beyond.

Freedom also no longer exists and has been exposed as a preprogrammed brain activity. This conclusion is based on Benjamin Libet's research, which shows that before the intention to perform an action from the brain, a signal is sent to the muscles (Libet, 1983). Apart from the methodology applied in his research, the premises of his experiment do not allow the conclusion that free will does not exist (Meynen, 2008). My impression is that Libet confuses two categories: free will and reflex.

Neuroscience tends to accommodate all human aspects in an all-encompassing physicalisation. The question is whether this position is tenable. Does this view make practical action better and easier? I think I have to doubt that given the massive dissatisfaction in mental health care among both workers and patients. It seems that humans are increasingly seen as neurophysiologically controlled machines whose behaviour is completely determined. He or she is an assembly of organs controlled by a neuronal network. Every shred of psychology and every claim to subjective freedom has been squeezed out of this model. This modern mindset is probably an offshoot of Enlightenment thinking. At the start of the Enlightenment, there were still a few who thought about man in physicalist terms, such as Julien Offray de La Mettrie, who saw man as a machine that could sometimes falter (La Mettrie, 1748). This idea has since become commonplace in large circles of psychiatry and beyond.

It is inevitable that such a view of people has consequences for the way patients are dealt with and treated. Signs of this are the immense increase in the prescription of psychotropic drugs to lubricate the machine and the frequent use of coercive measures to get the derailed machine back on track. Psychiatry is increasingly taking on a disciplining and surveillance character, despite the counter-movement of patient initiatives and of some professionals. Psychiatric practice in all its shades can ultimately be traced back to a view of man. Over the course of history, this view has shifted more and more towards an increasingly pervasive physicalist approach, which in fact has never disappeared in the existence of psychiatry but has become much more commonplace at the start of the third millennium.

Of course, there are also critical thinkers, but they have been marginalised as strange creatures who have little meaning in the world of psychiatry. The anti-psychiatric movement that took a critical stance towards the then current psychiatric practice is now fifty years behind us. I regularly ask mental health workers what foundations they base their daily work on, what kind of human image they use. They usually end up modifying or suppressing deviant behaviour and symptoms that are believed to be controlled by the derailed brain. The explanation is often that this is the result of evidence-based research. It is striking that many patients have adopted this view. Evidently, mechanistic thinking has become a cultural commonplace. When I object that these studies allow a delineated and limited window on reality and thereby exclude other areas, these alternative views are dismissed as unscientific. But then people forget that scientificity in psychiatry means that there must be a somatic substrate in psychiatric disorders. However, no such substrate is found in any of the disorders mentioned in the DSM-5, except when toxic substances are involved. But most poignantly, it is believed that there is no alternative. An alternative that leaves the church in the centre of the village, taking into account all aspects of the human being, in which both the psyche and the somatic have a place. In this regard, Engel's confession with its bio-psycho-social model is only a declaration of intent that should encourage a broader view of man (Engel, 1977). It is certainly not a model yet, but rather a reminder. This well-intentioned warning from Engel has failed to give psychiatric practice a solid theoretical foundation.

Unfortunately, in order to get a realistic view of man, we must not rely solely on medical science and for the past 75 years we no longer have to consult psychology, but rather have to resort to philosophy and then also be careful not to end up in the Anglo-Saxon waters, because the philosophers of that signature have a strong tendency to only reinforce the materialistic view. They excel in reasoning that is laced with language games in the context of logic, which seem imaginative and fun, but in fact go hand in hand. Think of Searle's "Chinese Room", the "Turing Test", "Brains in a Vat", "What is it like to be a Bat?" by Nagel and "Earth and Twin Earth" by Putnam. These thought experiments are very similar to the paradoxes formulated by Zeno of Elea; sterile constructs that eliminated part of reality leading to absurd conclusions. Think of the race between Achilles and the tortoise, which concluded that Achilles could not catch up with the tortoise.

John Searle, one of these somewhat critical Anglo-Saxon philosophers, found that his colleagues had engaged in the philosophy of mind for fifty years without realising that they were studying matters in the objective world without incorporating the subjective aspect involving the phenomenon of consciousness. In the footsteps of this philosophical discourse, psychological research has developed with the disastrous effect we are now left with. Searle found that the first-person ontology was approached in third-person terms (Searle, 1992, 95). With this, he put his finger on the sore spot that also concerns psychiatry and showed himself more nuanced than most of his Anglo-Saxon colleagues.

One of the most eloquent authors from the philosophical-materialist field is Daniel Dennett. In an accessible style, he argues that there is no basis for the psychic other than biology (Dennett, 1991). He admits that consciousness remains a mystery to materialists like himself, but he trusts that one day this mystery will be solved when someone rises and finds the key to this mystery somewhere in the brain. In this respect, he takes the same position as Freud, on the understanding that Freud has mainly described psychological mechanisms in his texts.[1] Dennett will continue to fight philosophical dualism *coûte que coûte*. Apparently, it is not necessary to observe something to know something for sure. Faith in it is enough.

In order to generate a more balanced view of man, it is better to stay in Europe and consult the phenomenologists and the psychoanalysts — not all — who recognise the difficulties surrounding the subject but take a more nuanced position in it than the Americans and some English realise. This study will mainly be based on structuralism, a philosophical direction with many extensions to fields other than philosophy, including psychiatry, with an emphasis on contextual-structuring moments for the subject.

What I have in mind in this publication is to bring out the potential creativity of nothingness. Everything starts with nothing. The subject is also born out of nothing. Nothingness gives the subject an almost supernatural power to start life and make something of it. This active force is difficult to name and is often referred to in vague terms according to the ideology adhered to by its author: *élan vital*, vital force, libido, drive, desire, and so on. In fact, one does not know what drives man. Scientists look for it but do not find it. Here and there it is mentioned with great aplomb that they have found it, but it soon becomes apparent that these authors have become entangled in their own ideology.

The life force has more to do with the nothing than with the something. The subject appears just like that and attaches itself to illusions and words in order to provide itself with something to hold on to, and in that movement, a person with a certain identity emerges. The subject manifests itself in doing and speaking. These are, of course, only activities to fill the void of nothingness. That stuffing is in fact not something that is tangible. The word is only an indication of something and therefore not a thing. It dissipates the moment it is spoken. But it does leave a trace. Traces in reality and traces in consciousness. These traces are of vital importance to the subject. It cannot live without these traces. Without these traces, it finds itself in a void that is unbearable. In the clinic, we recognise this in psychosis. Sometimes patients get close to this void and then become depressed and suicidal. During the Covid-19 pandemic, I have seen this on several occasions with young people who are in the process of inventing themselves and for that, they need more than others to mirror themselves and talk to each other. Due to the pandemic, they are forced to live in isolation and the Other is not or too little present.

In this text, I want to show what nothingness does to the subject and if there is no reaction to this, there is no subject formation. The clinic shows what disastrous consequences that can have. I will try to sketch the place and meaning of nothingness using metaphors such as the physical phenomenon of precipitation in the condensation vessel and Lacan's grapheme. In addition, my clinical experiences with patients who have come into contact with nothingness are extensively discussed. The manifestations of this are seen in the negative hallucination, the doppelgänger delusion, and Cotard's syndrome.

In this book, a view of man will be presented that does more justice to reality in a model in which the psychic in all its complex shades will be involved, while the somatic will not be lost sight of. Structuralism and linguistics will occupy an important place here because they expressly assign a place to the context of the subject, thereby avoiding a solipsistic view of man, a view of man that has forced psychiatry to look for a spirit in the body that, moreover, has never been found. Those who say they have found it have not searched properly (Kopland, 1972).

The model presented here is partly based on experiences from the clinic, where the negative plays a role, such as in the syndromes of Cotard and Capgras and the negative hallucination. They set us on the trail of the development of the subject, which experiences a void in separation that must be filled. This filling of the void that has arisen consists of imaginary and symbolic phenomena that cannot be traced back to material matters.

This study aims to illuminate the relationship between inside and outside that determine the structure of the subject. It is not for nothing that the symbol of Hermes, the god of the connection between the inside and the outside. He also has other names such as 'Strophaios', Hinge Point and 'Proturaios', Guardian, literally 'Before the Door'. He is a man, mobile, ruler of language and roads, messenger, master of messages, of interpretation, of communication and their ambiguities (Herter, 1976). He is also referred to as the soul's guide to the underworld (Rohde, 1893, 1925). Let Hermes be our guide in this quest for the subject in psychiatry.

This book argues for a rehabilitation of the subject. However, the subject escapes the objectifying ideology of science. It seems that object and subject are enemies. That should not be the case and in fact it is not, for the simple reason that in man the objective and the subjective come together. They maintain a dialectical relationship with each other. In the clinic, we can observe this daily, in particular with psychosomatic disorders.

The study of the subject has not existed for very long. In fact, this interest in the subject is made concrete with the adage of René Descartes *"je pense donc je suis"* (I think therefore I am). The subject is placed at the centre of thought. That was not the case in the Middle Ages. At that time, the individual was part of the collective whole that focused its gaze mainly on the transcendental, the higher. Since then, man's gaze has been directed more inward, resulting in a temporary (?) delay or end point in psychoanalysis. With the mechanisation of the human image, a countermovement seems to have arisen. In my view, this is a form of mental regression in Western culture. Against this, only a defence of the subject can be deployed.

However, the problem arises here that the subject has no ground, that is to say, the subject is not built up from matter where the substrate of the subject would be found. The subject is fundamentally separated from its origin, separated from its physical existence. The subject is a split being with a defect, a shortcoming. He no longer knows what he lacks because it disappeared during the primal repression. That is the nothingness that this book is constantly about. The nothingness cannot be observed but manifests itself in people's behaviour and experiences, in its symptoms.

Note

1 In his *Entwurf einer Psychologie*, Freud took an unadulterated biological view of the psychic mechanism. He never wanted to publish this pamphlet. It later became known because it was part of his correspondence with Wilhelm Fliess, published by Jeffrey Masson in 1950 (Freud, 1895). Later in his works he regularly referred to this biologistic point of view; it has always remained a longing for a biological or scientific foundation of psychoanalysis, he has never found a proof for this.

1

OUTLINE OF THE PROBLEM FACING PSYCHIATRY

Modern psychiatry faces significant challenges in addressing serious mental illnesses effectively. Psychological explanations are increasingly being replaced by naturalistic models. Symptoms are no longer interpreted or understood but are instead treated as nuisances to be eradicated. While phenomenology and psychoanalysis continue to explore the hermeneutic value of symptoms, they play only a minimal role in contemporary psychiatry.

Symptoms are inherently multifaceted and cannot be fully understood through either a purely somatic or psychological perspective. Both phenomenologically distinct dimensions must be acknowledged to achieve meaningful and effective treatment, particularly in psychiatry. Today, however, symptoms are disproportionately viewed through a somatic lens, often to the detriment of their psychological significance. To preserve the psychological dimension in psychiatry, far greater emphasis must be placed on the hermeneutic aspect of symptoms. Reducing all psychopathology to somatic explanations is not a solution. The psychological operates on a fundamentally different level, yet it is increasingly neglected, especially in academic settings.

The subject must be brought back into focus by mental health researchers and practitioners. However, this is a challenging endeavor because the tools necessary to address the problem have largely been lost. Those who engage with issues of subjectivity are often found not within psychiatry or psychology but among philosophers—who, more often than not, speak an entirely different language.

DOI: 10.4324/9781003675389-3

Psychiatry has yet to determine how to address the status of the psychological aspects of humanity. Consequently, it resorts to rigorous reductionism, supported and reinforced by brain research. This research rests on the premise that human behavior is merely a by-product of brain function. Such reasoning is circular, excluding other perspectives and yielding nothing more than a limited view of humanity. The impact of this reductionism on clinical practice is evident. Over the past 30 years, psychiatry has seen a tremendous increase in instrumental treatment methods, a significant rise in the consumption of psychotropic drugs, and the monopolization of behavioral therapy. The mechanization of psychiatry is further supported by a diagnostic system that categorizes deviant behavior in a way that aligns seamlessly with this reductive framework.

It seems that psychiatry is losing control of its core business, the treatment of psychoses. This powerlessness is evident, for example, from the increase in the number of compulsory admissions, while they wanted to reduce them. Several authors who are intensively involved in the treatment of psychosis are watching this development with dismay (Vanheule, 2013, 2023).

It is undeniable that modern psychiatry increasingly relies on judicial support to work with patients who have not sought treatment themselves. Whether new legislation for psychiatry—such as the *Wvggz* (Compulsory Mental Health Act) and the *Wzd* (Wet Zorg en Dwang, or Care and Coercion Act)—will bring meaningful change remains to be seen (*WvS*, 2020). Psychiatry appears to be taking on a surveillance role, aiming to rid society of troublesome or confused individuals who do not conform to societal norms. The social function of psychiatry is becoming increasingly dominant, often at the expense of liberating patients from their psychopathological prisons. The group takes precedence over the individual; society over the citizen.

Not long ago, phenomenological psychiatry flourished in the Netherlands, playing a prominent international role in the field. Psychoanalysis, too, had a major influence on psychiatric theory and treatment methods during the latter half of the 20th century. Both approaches gave significant attention to the psychic dimension without neglecting the physical. Yet both have almost entirely disappeared from psychiatric practice, dismissed as unscientific.

What remains is a system focused on symptom management and modification, characterized by a strongly instrumental approach. The market-driven forces institutionalized across healthcare fit neatly with the control mechanisms that now dominate psychiatry. Processes are streamlined and executed efficiently. Every detail of healthcare is scrutinized by health insurers. Everything appears to be under control. However, the reality is far from this. Control mechanisms have reached their limits. Rebellious behavior is becoming increasingly common, and dissatisfaction is pervasive. Little seems to have changed since Freud wrote *Civilisation and Its Discontents* (*Das Unbehagen in der Kultur*) near the end of his life (Freud, 1930/1961). Crime, terrorism, and drug use have now taken on extreme forms.

The need for new techniques to maintain control has led to a crisis, exacerbated by the absence of an adequate theoretical foundation. Humanity does not easily relinquish its freedom, even when acting thoughtlessly. Psychiatry's greatest problem, one that has persisted for centuries, remains the mind–body dualism. This issue can be traced back to Cartesian dualism, though it has evolved in various forms. Current views in psychiatry and psychological philosophy lean heavily toward unadulterated materialism, often referred to as naturalism. Monistic determinism is almost universally accepted in psychiatry, aligning with the tendencies characteristic of Anglo-Saxon philosophy of mind.

Fortunately, within this philosophical and conceptual framework, there are critical perspectives that challenge this one-sided materialism. For instance, David Chalmers has offered a more balanced critique. Prominent proponents of psychological physicalism include Hilary Putnam and Paul Churchland, each contributing distinct interpretations (Putnam, 1981; Churchland, 1981). Daniel Dennett, while adopting a more nuanced position, ultimately remains within the framework of materialistic monism (Dennett, 1991).

Thomas Nagel, however, firmly rejects psychological physicalism, arguing that it cannot account for the psychic in physical terms (Nagel, 1974). His critique extends to the inherent contradiction between the subjective and the objective. Materialists regard the objective as the sole foundation of science, reducing all psychic phenomena and subjective experiences to physical mechanisms. Nagel, however, contends that the transition from the subjective to the objective has insurmountable limits. He argues that understanding the subjective would require a higher form of intelligence than humans possess: "The subjective domain in all its qualities implies the belief in the existence of facts beyond the reach of human concepts" (Nagel, 1974, p. 532).

Nagel's perspective suggests the existence of a vertical transcendence. However, in my view, such transcendence is unnecessary for modelling subject dualism. A more grounded approach, akin to Sartre's *La transcendence de l'ego* (Sartre, 1936), may be sufficient.

The Mind–Body Problem and the Subjective Experience

A common feature among monistic reductionists is their tendency to regard the psychic and the physical as identical. They attempt to solve the mind–body problem by obscuring the independent status of the mind, akin to cutting the Gordian knot. However, it is challenging to reconcile what is meant by the "objective nature" of an experience that fundamentally belongs to the private realm of subjective experience. For instance, when brain processes are made visible through imaging techniques, the subjective experience accompanying these processes remains inaccessible. The subject must articulate their experience, which another person might approximately recognize—a point emphasized by Karl Jaspers in the first footnote[1] of *General Psychopathology*. However, the "other" must rely on their own subjective experiences to interpret those of the subject, highlighting the inherent gap between subjective and objective understanding. Even with advanced empathy, the other remains an outsider to another's subjective realm.

As tools to explore the brain become increasingly sophisticated, monistic reductionists argue that subjective phenomena will come closer to being objectively understood. This reasoning, however, is illusory. It can be likened to a positive hallucination—perceiving something that isn't there—or perhaps a negative hallucination, where the subjective experience is removed from view. Either way, this interpretive error borders on delusion. Negative hallucinations are discussed in Chapter 9 in relation to one of three clinical vignettes.

In psychiatric practice, the exchange of experiences is mediated through language, enabling a symbolic connection to objective reality. Words clarify and communicate, but they are also subject to misinterpretation. Furthermore, subjects themselves rely on the symbolic order of language to signify their identity and make sense of their consciousness. In doing so, they encounter the inherent limitations of language. As Michel Foucault (1963) observed, the symbolic order of words never fully corresponds to the things they signify. This fascinating yet complex subject will be explored further in Chapter 5.

Physicalists assert that mental phenomena are merely physical phenomena. Yet no evidence has substantiated this hypothesis. Proponents argue that evidence will emerge in the future, but the subjective nature of experience presents a significant obstacle to this claim. Until validated, this assertion remains an axiom without scientific support and must be rejected.

Mind and body belong to fundamentally different epistemological orders. Equating them without acknowledgment of their distinct properties distorts their understanding. Thus, the mind–body problem persists as an unresolved enigma. Treating the mind and body as equivalent is a speculative leap inconsistent with the principles of objective science.

There are, however, models that provide a more nuanced view of the interaction between the psychic and the physical. Yet these too confront inherent limitations, which will be discussed.

In this study, structuralism serves as a foundation for examining the highly complex nature of humanity. Phenomenology and psychoanalysis are referenced to complement this framework, as both acknowledge the heterogeneous composition of human experience. Phenomenology investigates phenomena in their meanings and suspends judgment (*episteme*), while psychoanalysis delves into the dynamics between conscious and unconscious processes. Structuralism integrates these perspectives, incorporating the somatic aspect of the Real into a cohesive framework.

Structuralism's orientation contrasts sharply with Anglo-Saxon philosophy and traces its roots to Ferdinand de Saussure's linguistics. A more detailed examination of structuralism's contributions will follow in Chapter 4.

Note

1 "The word *phenomenology* is from Hegel used for the totality of the appearances of the spirit in consciousness, history and thought. We need it for the much narrower area of individual mental experience. Husserl initially used the word for 'descriptive psychology' of the phenomena of consciousness—in this sense, it applies to our investigations—but later for 'essential vision' (*Wesensschau*), which we do not pursue here. Only here is phenomenology an empirical experience; it is kept going solely by the fact that the *patient communicates it* (*Mitteilung seitens des Kranken*). It is obvious that this psychological procedure is different from that of scientific descriptions: the object itself is not sensuous to our eyes, since experience is only visualization. But the logical principle is no different. Describing requires, besides systematic categories, fortunate formulations and contrasting comparisons, marking the understanding of phenomena, their order in series, or their occurrence in seamless leaps" (Jaspers, 1913, p. 47). (translation JdK).

2

HISTORICAL DEVELOPMENT OF PSYCHIATRY FROM THE ENLIGHTENMENT

In this study on the mechanization of psychiatry and its difficulties, we will not attempt to outline its entire history but will focus on the aspects that are most relevant to our subject. Naturally, we take the Enlightenment as our starting point, as modern thinking is fundamentally rooted in this era. Structuralism provides a key critique of Enlightenment thinking, with Michel Foucault as one of its most important figures. Foucault's critique, centered on the concept of power, offers particularly valuable insights for understanding contemporary psychiatry.

However, the question arises as to whether Foucault is the best guide in our search for the subject. He was, above all, a thinker of power and had a unique understanding of its exercise within psychiatry. For Foucault, power was primarily external, imposed by the Other, and his critique rarely addressed internal dynamics of power, such as those within the subject or in relation to the unconscious.

Other critics of psychiatry have also focused predominantly on its institutional aspects. Thomas Szasz argued that psychiatry was primarily an institution of control, aimed at managing deviant behavior for reasons unrelated to science. Eugen Bleuler, on the other hand, suggested that medicine—and psychiatry in particular—was too inward-looking to contribute anything meaningful to society, let alone to its patients.

In all these critiques, the subjective dimension was neglected, leaving a significant gap in the discourse on psychiatry and its practices.

Foucault's first major publication concerns psychiatry. In his *History of Madness*, he examines a certain aspect of Western society during the transition from the Middle Ages to the Renaissance (Foucault, 1963).

DOI: 10.4324/9781003675389-4

He describes in detail the way we deal with "senseless people," which, due to chance circumstances, takes a completely different turn than was previously the case. According to Foucault, the individual (read: the subject)[1] did not yet exist at all in this period; he only appeared on the scene at the transition to the 19th century.[2] Before that time, culture was mainly dominated by concepts such as God, the world, the likeness of things, and the laws of space, and there was also great attention for the bodies, passions, and imagination. "But man himself is completely absent from this" (Bonnefoi, 1966).

Foucault was deeply influenced by Nietzsche's reading, not only in terms of power but also in his deep-seated awareness of the historicity of the origins of human habits. Consider *Also sprach Zarathustra* (*Thus Spoke Zarathustra*) (Nietzsche, 1885) and *Zur Genealogie der Moral* (On the Genealogy of Morals) (Nietzsche, 1887). Like Nietzsche, Foucault arrives at an analysis of power as a normal human phenomenon and not as a perversely pathological outgrowth of human behavior (Foucault, 1969). This does not alter the fact that there is such a thing as the abuse of power.

Foucault paints a bleak picture of the future human being who, through all kinds of manipulations of collected data and an insatiable control compulsion, will make humans evolve into a zombie that will only be short-lived. He will disappear into a black hole that he has dug for himself. His freedom and his desires will be taken from him because all his needs will be satisfied. Needs dictated by the media, which will play an even greater role than they already assume. From an evolutionary point of view, man will adapt to a passionless way of existence that lacks any form of creativity.

According to Foucault, power is not a state monopoly but rather an ingredient of the culture that we all shape together. Something is shifting in the view of life and the role that humans play in it. One aspect of this is that having takes precedence over being. This concerns not only the possession of material things but also qualities such as those in psychiatry, which come to the fore when expressions such as "I have depression, autism, or ADHD" are used. These qualifications have come about through "scientifically sound research methods" and are communicated to us by an authority in this field: the psychiatrist. More and more use is made of techniques and control systems that determine the actual power. The increase in means of communication and the pandemic spread of the influence of the media are examples of this. Power is no longer attributable to an enlightened or unenlightened despot or the state. Power is a kind of virus that roams the culture and kills people who, in all freedoms, allow themselves to be seduced by the media without their noticing. Some media are consciously manipulating, and others are not, because they assume they are doing the right thing. The media assume that their activities only promote progress, and those who are manipulated find that their wants and needs are met. The paradox arises that this power play is at the expense of individual freedom and the extinction of creativity.

It seems that psychiatric patients are evading this game, but that's an illusion. Psychiatry is also a participant in this game, for both patients and professionals. Sometimes it does indeed appear that patients are not playing the game by rebelling against the treatment regimen, for example, when patients do not get better despite all efforts in applying treatment techniques or when they actually resist, but the latter is really just the psychotic and probably not for much longer, because it has already come to the point that he adopts his diagnosis "schizophrenia" and even asks for medication, which was certainly not the case some 50 years ago.

It is to be hoped that Foucault is wrong in his vision of the future and that his analysis of the power play contributes to its countermovement so that the subject does not die out like footsteps disappearing in the sand at the edge of the sea[3] (Foucault, 1968). The Foucauldian view of power and manipulation has found little resonance in psychiatry. Psychiatrists regard him as an outsider who cannot have a say in the reality of the psychiatric field. This criticism is unjustified because the position of the outsider is necessary in order to be able to withdraw from the dominant discourse in psychiatry. Professionals are often blinded by their status as physicians who want the best for patients. Foucault's publications make us think, and we need a listening ear.

Innovations in psychiatry usually do not come from the professionals. Rather, they hammer at the same anvil of psychic physicalism. That makes a lot of noise, but little music comes out of it.

What Michel Foucault has in common with almost all structuralists is that he denies belonging to this group of thinkers. Yet there are indications in his texts that do point in the direction of structuralism. Constantly emphasizing the subject's decentralized status is part of this. Despite his denial, it is common practice to classify Foucault as part of the structuralist movement within philosophy (Kwant, 1978).

In his philosophy, Foucault has mainly concerned himself with the status of knowledge, constantly resisting the subject-centralist thinking of knowledge in Western philosophy, culminating in Hegel's all-encompassing philosophy. Initially interested in historical matters in which certain structures in society changed, such as insane asylums, hospitals, and prisons, he later focused on an analysis of knowledge itself and the role that power plays in it, resulting in a three-part analysis of sexuality (Foucault, 1976–2018). All three are, of course, also subject to structural changes. In his *Archéologie du savoir*, Foucault is entirely interested in knowing that has become separated from subjective knowledge. In fact, he then takes the position that is closely related to that of the natural sciences (Foucault, 1969). Yet he does not target knowledge of matter but rather knowledge as knowing, the discourse of knowledge. In that sense, he is a true philosopher and not a scientist.

Here there is a big difference with structuralist psychoanalysis, where the focus is mainly on the individual, the particularity of the subjective experience, you could say the *parole* (speech, word). The contradiction seems to be very great, but in practice it is not too bad when one considers that psychoanalysis is also concerned with general knowledge and the *langue* (language).[4] Moreover, Foucault cannot ignore the fact that knowledge can only be expressed and experienced through the subject.

Foucault's style is quite provocative and is characterized by a resistance to everything and everyone, but he can also change his point of view later. He called himself a philosopher but was also intensively involved in fields such as psychiatry, medicine, linguistics, psychology, and sociology. He always analyzed these areas with William Ockham's razor and interpreted the changes therein as fractures at the level of epistemic conditions (Karskens, 1986). He was no stranger to moralistic and critical attitudes toward social and cultural customs. One could say that he has adopted Nietzsche's moralistic whip.

His attitude to psychoanalysis was initially positive because it would tie in with the counter-science that could break through the modern episteme (Karskens, 1986). Later, he opposed psychoanalysis because it would not lead to scientific knowledge. In a similar way, he dealt with the phenomenology he so admired in Binswanger, but he rejected this mindset for quite the same reason as he did psychoanalysis. He vehemently opposed the falseness of the human sciences and saw it as his task to expose them. Psychology and psychiatry, in particular, had to bear the brunt of this.

Whence this fierceness? After all, he was an outsider to these fields. He only studied and criticized psychology and psychiatry from texts and not from contacts with patients and psychotherapists, I assume. His critical fervor is remarkable. One would almost assume that he suffered a trauma in this area at some point in his life. This does not alter the fact that his criticism makes sense and forms a good counterbalance to a cold, objectifying psychiatric practice that is spreading at the beginning of the 21st century.

The fact that many psychoanalysts in recent decades have strongly leaned toward a scientific foundation of psychoanalysis is based not only on Freud's *Entwurf* (Freud, 1895) but also on regular expressions of his wish to one day see that psychological mechanisms are organic pillars. Two quotes can show that:

> Thirdly, it must be borne in mind that all our psychological assumptions must one day be founded on organic pillars. It will probably then become apparent that there are special substances and chemical processes that sort out the effects of sexuality and ensure the continuation of individual life within that of the species. We take this probability into account by substituting special chemical substances for special psychic powers.
>
> *(Freud, 1914)*

and:

> Precisely because I always try to protect psychology from every other kind of thinking, including biological thinking, I want to expressly acknowledge here that the hypothesis of separate ego and sexual drives, i.e., the libido theory, rests by no means on a psychological basis and is essentially biologically based. I will therefore also be consistent in dropping this hypothesis as soon as psychoanalytic practice itself reveals a different and more useful premise about drives. That has not been the case until now.
>
> *(Freud, 1914)*

The desire to have a biological foundation for psychological processes emerges from these quotations, and this is also expressed in Freud's choice of words when speaking of drives, which have such a clear biological connotation. So in all Freud's references to this theme of a material foundation of psychic processes, there is a wish for which he, too, was unable to put forward any facts. In the meantime, he has developed a very elaborate and nuanced model of the psyche that is not biologically based.

The criticism of psychiatry does not only come from outside; mechanistic thinking in both psychiatry and psychoanalysis has also been criticized from within.

The critics from within are to be feared the most. Just think of Martin Luther, whose criticism of the abuses in the Catholic Church gave rise to a schism. In psychiatry, one can think of Thomas Szasz, who bombarded psychiatry with pamphlet after pamphlet with fundamental criticism of the scientific claim of this specialism. He even called the idea of madness an error similar to the madness itself (Szasz, 1961). A group that is generally negative toward psychiatry is also the patients, and especially the patients who are confronted with compulsory admission.

In the last century, well before the 1960s and 1970s, the psychiatrist Eugen Bleuler occasionally criticized medicine in general, but this critical publication has had little impact. The title of this book was not tender, and the content did not lie. Thinking in medicine would have turned in on itself and that would stand in the way of scientific development. Bleuler also saw a possibility of escaping the shortcoming of a monothetic somatic orientation. Despite the remarkable title *Das autistisch-undiziplinierte Denken in der Medizin und seine Überwindung* ("The Autistic-Undisciplined Thinking in Medicine and Its Solution"), it has found little resonance in medical circles and also not in psychiatry, while Bleuler was nevertheless at the time an authority in those circles and even a celebrity for coining the term "schizophrenia" (Bleuler, 1919).

Notes

1 The word individual comes from the Latin *individuum*, not divisible. Before modern times, man was part of the group that made up society and had little significance as a separate person. He or she was the indivisible element of the group. From the seventeenth century, the term individual took on the meaning of a separate element, whereby the commonality of the group came more into the background and individualism was born. Later we will see in Descartes and Lacan that the subject is shared, but in both thinkers in a different way; *res extensa* and *res cogitans* in Descartes and in Lacan the *sujet barré*, the barred subject in which the individual enters into the symbolic order and thereby distances himself from a part of himself, from his own body.

2 Later, in his *The order of Things*, Foucault will even assume that the subject has already disappeared (Foucault, 1966).

3 Perhaps Foucault was inspired in his imagery by a poem by Jacques Prévert, *Les feuilles mortes (Autumn leaves)*: Mais la vie sépare ceux qui s'aiment,/ Tout doucement sans faire de bruit/ Et la mer efface sur le sable/ Les pas des amants désunis (But life separates those who love each other/slowly and quietly/and the sea erases on the sand/the steps of the disunited lovers).

4 *Parole* and *langue* are aspects of the language in which *parole* represents individual language utterances, concrete speech and *langue* concerns the structure of the language system. I will return to these aspects later in Chapter 4.

PART 2

Structuralism and Nothingness

Introduction

Structuralism, a seminal intellectual movement of the 20th century, emerged from the pioneering linguistic work of Ferdinand de Saussure, whose *Cours de Linguistique Générale* laid the foundation for a profound rethinking of meaning, language, and the subject. This school of thought has significantly influenced fields as diverse as anthropology, psychoanalysis, philosophy, literature, and the human sciences, while also intersecting with ongoing debates concerning the nature of subjectivity and the implications of *nothingness* for human thought and creativity.At the heart of Saussure's theory lies the concept of the linguistic sign, composed of the *signifier* (sound or written form) and the *signified* (concept or meaning). Importantly, these two elements are not naturally connected; rather, their relationship is arbitrary and relational, which implies that meaning arises not from intrinsic connections but through differences within a system.

Saussure's distinction between *langue* (the structured, shared language system) and *parole* (individual speech acts) became a cornerstone of structuralist analysis. Langue is collective and rule-governed, whereas parole is individual and fluid. The systematic study of langue allows one to comprehend the abstract mechanisms by which meaning is generated, whereas parole reflects the personal and creative use of language.

While structuralism originated in linguistics, it quickly migrated into other disciplines. Figures such as Claude Lévi-Strauss in anthropology, Jacques Lacan in psychoanalysis, Michel Foucault in philosophy and the history of ideas, and Roland Barthes in literary theory expanded the

DOI: 10.4324/9781003675389-5

structuralist method to analyse cultural systems, power relations, and the formation of the subject.

One of the most significant shifts these thinkers introduced was a rejection of essentialism—the belief that meaning or identity stems from a fixed inner core or transcendent truth. Instead, they emphasised the primacy of structure: identity and meaning are produced through differences and oppositions embedded in systems of signs. This perspective parallels Heidegger's notion in *Der Satz vom Grund* that being has no secure ground, and meaning arises from relational configurations rather than foundational truths (Heidegger, 1956–1957).

In the field of psychoanalysis, Lacan reinterpreted Freud through the lens of structuralism, particularly Saussure's ideas. He famously reversed Saussure's hierarchy, arguing that the signifier precedes the signified, thus positioning language as the primary force in shaping the unconscious and the subject.

For Lacan, entry into the symbolic order—the domain of language, law, and social norms—constitutes a fundamental break in the development of the subject. The mirror stage, in which the child recognises its reflection as a unified image, is the first moment of alienation, initiating a split within the self that is never fully resolved. The symbolic order imposes meaning, but always imperfectly, leaving behind a residue of lack—what Lacan calls the Real—which resists symbolization.

The theme of nothingness—explored in Greek philosophy and developed in modern thought by thinkers like Kant and Heidegger—is reintroduced in this context as a productive gap or lack inherent to subjectivity and language. The split between word and thing, between symbol and referent, is not merely a limitation but a constitutive absence that gives rise to thought, desire, and the subject itself.

In the early development of the child, the separation from the mother produces a void—a loss or castration, in Lacanian terms—that language attempts to mediate. Yet words, too, are based on nothing; they do not correspond directly to reality. This fundamental impossibility underpins the process of symbolization, which is crucial for the emergence of consciousness, identity, and relationality.

The developmental psychology of Henri Wallon, which influenced Lacan, provides insight into how children begin to differentiate themselves from others. In the mirror stage, the child encounters itself as an external image, experiencing both unity and alienation. The child's developing self-awareness depends on creating a distance—not only from the physical mother but also from its own fragmented body.

This distance recurs throughout symbolic development: perception requires detachment; symbolization requires separation. Language inserts a gap between subject and object, enabling abstraction, memory, and imagination. Thus, subjectivity is not grounded in continuity or fullness but in division, loss, and lack.

Lacan's conception of the *sujet barré* (barred subject) encapsulates this divided nature of the self. The subject is alienated from itself and exists only through its symbolic representations. Every word spoken signifies not presence but absence—a missing fullness that can never be recovered.

Science, with its orientation towards objectivity, measurability, and clarity, struggles with concepts such as nothingness, subjectivity, and the Real. Structuralism—and Lacanian theory in particular—offers a powerful critique of the reductive tendencies of scientific discourse, especially within psychiatry and psychology.

Modern science, especially in the wake of positivism, marginalises the role of the subject in favour of observable data. Yet figures such as Heisenberg, with his uncertainty principle, have demonstrated that observation is always mediated by the observer, and thus subjectivity cannot be eliminated from the equation.

In fields like psychiatry, this objectivist approach leads to a reliance on biological models and statistical norms, at the expense of understanding the symbolic, imaginative, and relational dimensions of mental life. The resurgence of biological psychiatry is thus seen as a defensive reaction to the challenges posed by structuralist and post-structuralist thought.

Despite its seemingly negative connotations, nothingness is not merely an absence; it is a generative space—the site of desire, creativity, and symbolic invention. The gap between word and thing opens up a space in which new meanings can emerge, through imagination, metaphor, and poetic expression.

This idea has far-reaching implications. Language, far from being a flawed tool, becomes the very condition for freedom and creativity. Its structure allows for an infinite play of signifiers, making possible both scientific inquiry and artistic creation. The impossibility of closure—of ever fully representing reality—invites continuous reinterpretation and innovation.

Importantly, the symbolic does not resolve the gap between being and appearance; it sustains it, making room for the desire that animates human life. Desire, in Lacanian terms, is never fulfilled but is continuously redirected through speech and other symbolic acts.

The symbolic order, while enabling creativity, also holds a fragile structure. When it breaks down—as in psychosis—the distinction between reality and imagination can collapse. This collapse is evident in symptoms such as hallucinations and delusions, where the symbolic no longer provides a stable framework for meaning.

Nevertheless, this same symbolic instability allows for extraordinary artistic and intellectual achievements. Artists and poets often explore the edges of the symbolic order, giving form to the void and rendering visible what is normally invisible.

Thus, the symbolic gap is ambivalent: it is both the condition for subjectivity and its potential undoing. Structuralism, in revealing this ambivalence, challenges simplistic models of the mind and instead foregrounds the complex interplay of language, desire, and the unconscious.

Structuralism and its exploration of language, nothingness, and subjectivity represent a decisive break from earlier philosophical and scientific models. Rather than seeking to eliminate uncertainty, structuralism embraces it as the core of human experience.

The subject, far from being a stable, rational entity, is revealed as divided, desiring, and embedded in symbolic networks. Language does not mirror reality but constitutes it in ever-shifting ways. Nothingness, similarly, is not an abyss to be feared but a creative force that makes possible the richness of thought, speech, and human connection.

The challenge for disciplines such as psychiatry and psychology is to resist the lure of total objectivity and to reclaim the subjective, symbolic, and imaginative dimensions of the human condition. Structuralism, far from being outdated, continues to offer profound insights into the nature of meaning, identity, and reality.

As such, the legacy of Saussure, Lacan, and their successors remains vital for anyone concerned with understanding not only the mind but the structures and ruptures that shape our existence.

3
STRUCTURALISM

Structuralism began with Ferdinand de Saussure's *Cours de Linguistique Générale*, in which he studied the structure of language and formulated a theory about it. The most basic part of language is the sign, which he divided into the signified and the signifier, two distinct elements that maintain a relationship. This fundamental separation appears, in one form or another, in the ideas of all structuralists. Also originating from Saussure is the notion that a word only acquires meaning in relation to a context, just as the subject only acquires identity in relation to the Other in Lacan's theory.

The most famous structuralists are Lévi-Strauss, Foucault, Lacan, and Barthes. A relatively recent addition to this group is Bracha Ettinger, whose idea of the matrixial borderspace discusses a network of possible sexual identities.

What structuralists share is the idea that there is no foundational ground for meaning, as can also be observed in Heidegger's *Der Satz von Grund (The Principal of Ground, 1956, 1974)*. This view stems partly from their deviation from Saussure's representation of the sign, in which the signified was thought to take precedence over the signifier. This interpretation can be traced back to Plato's idea of a transcendental world containing the truth behind phenomena. Structuralists rejected this notion, instead prioritizing the signifier over the signified.

As a result, there is no essential foundation for the signifier, and meaning only emerges in the sequence of signifiers.

With the advent of structuralism in Western thought, an intriguing phenomenon emerged that highlights the essence of this school of thought. Structuralism has its roots in linguistics, and it would have been expected that

DOI: 10.4324/9781003675389-6

there would be no specific text or author to reference as its source. Nevertheless, the name Ferdinand de Saussure is associated with it, thanks to the diligence of some of his students.[1] As a professor of linguistics at the University of Geneva, he delivered lectures presenting a new perspective on linguistics—a linguistics distinct from the historical tradition. At that time, a different perspective on linguistics was already emerging among scholars, likely why Saussure did not consider it necessary to commit his thoughts to writing. This history demonstrates that new insights did not appear out of the blue but were already present *in statu nascendi* among his peers, while also underscoring that the development of these ideas was not the product of a single author. Nonetheless, Saussure's audience recognized something significant in his teachings, and some students compiled his *Cours de Linguistique Générale* based on lecture notes. It was only much later that Saussure's ideas gained wider recognition, providing a crucial impetus to structuralism. By the 1950s and 1960s, this movement, with figures like Claude Lévi-Strauss, Jean Piaget, Michel Foucault, and Jacques Lacan, had spread into fields as diverse as anthropology, psychology, philosophy, and psychoanalysis.

From the outset, Saussure emphasized that language cannot be separated from the individuals who speak it. Later, Lacan would highlight this aspect as a crucial factor in the therapeutic relationship with patients. When one asks what language is, the question may seem absurd and irrelevant because languages such as English clearly exist, but not without being tied to those who speak them. Saussure distinguishes between *langue* (language as an abstract system) and *parole* (speech, or the concrete use of language). Although intertwined, they are absolutely distinct. This strict separation is mirrored in structuralist thought, seen in works such as Foucault's *Les Mots et les Choses* (*The Order of Things*, 1966) and Lacan's theories of *scission* (split) and castration, which appear in several of his texts (Lacan, 1966).[2]

Langue is governed by grammar and syntax and possesses a canonical quality, while *parole* is fleeting, evading linguistic rules, and characterized by creativity and freedom. *Langue* is collective and enduring; *parole* is instantaneous and personal. Though intertwined, Saussure insists they must be studied separately. Studying *langue* involves focusing on a singular system or structure, whereas studying *parole* examines its variety.

Saussure justifies this distinction as follows:

> By assigning the science of the *langue* its true place within the whole of the study of language, we have suddenly summed up linguistics in its entirety. All other parts of the language, which together make up the *parole*, naturally add themselves to this first science, and thanks to this amalgamation all parts of linguistics find their natural place.

Changes in language originate in *parole* but only impact *langue* after a considerable period.

Saussure rejected nomenclature, the triangular relationship between word, concept, and thing. For example, while a word like "tree" fits this model, abstract words like "present" and prepositions like "in" or "through" do not. Thus, the relationship between word and thing is contingent. This fundamental separation between word and thing recurs in discussions of the subject entering the symbolic order and beginning to use language.

Saussure also argued that without signs, ideas cannot be clearly or permanently distinguished. Thoughts are like a nebulous cloud. Sounds and words only acquire meaning within a linguistic system.

In exploring the body–mind dialectic, Saussure's analysis of language offers insight into the challenges of psychiatry, particularly in disorders where physicalist approaches have reached a dead end. Monistic theories fail to capture the complexities of the human sciences, leading to inadequate practices. Saussure's work highlights the necessity of recognizing the symbolic nature of language and its limitations while appreciating its creative possibilities.

Saussure's revolutionary perspective, even during his lifetime, underlined the relationship between language and thought. He wrote: "In every state (*of langue*) the mind is breathed into a given material and brings it to life." Language is not material; its symbolic aspect transcends physicality.

Although Saussure placed the signified above the signifier, Lacan later reversed this priority to emphasize the immediacy of speech in the therapeutic process. For Saussure, both the signified and the signifier exist within the psychic domain, comparable to Plato's idea, yet remain abstract. Mathematics provides a helpful analogy: while mathematical terms have signifieds, they are not demonstrable realities but abstract concepts.

To clarify these ideas, music serves as a useful comparison. *Langue* is akin to a piano, with its mechanisms and structure, while *parole* is like a piano sonata, performed with expressiveness unique to the musician.

Contingency plays a vital role in the relationship between signifier and signified, as Saussure explains. Symbolization, crucial for forming identity, relies on this contingent relationship, underscoring our dependence on the Other. Memory, too, plays an essential role in maintaining this relationship.

Structuralism profoundly influenced disciplines like sociology, history, linguistics, psychology, and cinema, though psychiatry has largely ignored it due to its alignment with medical sciences. This can largely be attributed to the medicalization of psychiatry, which prioritizes materialistic and biological explanations over symbolic or relational understandings of mental phenomena. The dominance of natural science paradigms has marginalized the contributions of structuralism and similar schools of thought.

Historically, psychiatry's focus on the somatic aspects of mental illness has fluctuated in response to cultural and intellectual movements. The resurgence of biological psychiatry in the late 20th century can be seen as a reaction to the perceived excesses of antipsychiatry, which aligned more closely with structuralist and post-structuralist ideas. However, this somatic revival has led to an oversimplification of complex human experiences and a neglect of the symbolic dimensions of mental health.

In contrast, structuralist approaches offer a richer understanding of the interplay between internal and external realities. By highlighting the relational nature of meaning and identity, structuralism provides tools for addressing the fragmented experiences of individuals in modern society. For example, the concept of *extimacy*—the intertwining of internal and external realities—captures the porous boundaries between the self and the Other. This idea resonates with the ancient Greek understanding of the relationship between the individual and the community, as seen in the polis and the agora.

Structuralism's emphasis on relationality challenges the self-contained, individualistic view of modernity. Instead, it underscores the ways in which our identities and experiences are shaped by interactions with others. This perspective has profound implications for disciplines such as sociology, history, and psychology, as well as for broader cultural and philosophical debates.

By moving away from denotative thinking, structuralism has opened up new possibilities for exploring the fluidity of meaning and the complexity of human relationships. The connotative approach allows for a multiplicity of interpretations and a more nuanced understanding of the human condition. However, this freedom comes with the recognition that meaning is always contingent and subject to change. Structuralism thus invites us to embrace the uncertainty and creativity inherent in the process of meaning-making.

In conclusion, structuralism has had a transformative impact on Western thought, reshaping our understanding of language, identity, and meaning. While its influence on certain fields, such as psychiatry, has been limited, its contributions to the humanities and social sciences remain profound. By challenging traditional notions of stability and certainty, structuralism has paved the way for new ways of thinking and being in the world. Its legacy continues to inspire scholars and practitioners to explore the intricate interplay between structure and freedom, the self and the Other, and the symbolic and the real.

Notes

1 Charles Bally, Albert Sechehaye, and Albert Riedlinger, who edited "Cours de Linguistique Générale" (1916).

2 Lacan used the term *castration* to refer to the separation between mother and child. He used this powerful expression to emphasize the traumatic and irrevocable nature of this event. *Scission* (split) is related to *castration* and concerns the separation within the becoming subject itself, where, entering into the symbolic order, the subject distances himself from a part of himself, from the Real of which the body is a part. Through this event, the child can begin to signify itself and acquire its own identity.

4

FUNDAMENTAL IMPOSSIBILITIES

The concept of nothingness has its origins in early Greek philosophy, beginning with Parmenides and continuing through Kant and Heidegger. Nothingness relates intrinsically to being, an ideal we never fully achieve. Desire, the force bridging the gap between being and existence (Dasein), perpetuates this dynamic tension. From an Aristotelian perspective, the subject arises without a material cause but has an efficient cause, as evidenced by the effects it produces despite the absence of a discernible object.

Psychogenesis begins with the separation between mother and child where a gap arises that needs to be filled. This is done with words that also ensure that consciousness can arise. The first relationship between the becoming subject and the Other proceeds along the mirror stage and is later symbolically filled in with words. There always remains a fundamental space between word and thing, despite what modern materialistic monism would have us believe.

The emptiness that arises in separation, also called "castration" by Lacan, installs nothingness in the subject and this nothingness continues in the use of words because words in fact also refer to nothing. Words are based on nothing, they have no ground. Only in their mutual difference can they generate meaning. From nothingness the subject creates a self that is actually an imaginary creation.

When we broach the subject of fundamental impossibilities, I do not immediately think of the perhaps unsolvable problem of the mind–body contradiction, but rather of the impossibility of the Real. Nevertheless, one is related to the other. Following Lacan, the Real is denoted as that which lies beyond the reach of the Symbolic. This might appear to be a

DOI: 10.4324/9781003675389-7

catastrophic condition, but it is, in fact, a sine qua non for the subject. To understand this, some explanation is necessary. The best way to elucidate this difficult point in Lacan's teaching is to reflect on the development of the young child in relation to the mother. In doing so, the psychological birth of the subject may come to light. The phases of the mirror stage and the transition to symbolization play an essential role in this process. In both events—mirroring and symbolizing—distance is an integral part of the subject's emergence. To perceive oneself in a mirror, one must create a distance, enabling a view of oneself. While this seems self-evident, in practice we rarely give it much thought. In symbolizing, a similar dynamic occurs as with mirroring, but it is more challenging to imagine because it is abstract in nature. Symbolization essentially takes place through language. In speaking, one distances oneself from reality. The word does not coincide with the object it signifies. There exists an impossibility between word and object, which nonetheless—or perhaps precisely because of this—supports the process of symbolization. Without this fundamental impossibility between word and object, there would be no need to symbolize.

To better understand these two faculties of humanity—perception and symbolization—it is helpful to consider the development of the young child. For this, we take as a starting point the behavior of the child in front of a mirror as described by Henri Wallon, a French developmental psychologist, whose publications informed Lacan's concept of the mirror stage (Wallon, 1949).

The psychological birth of the subject is preceded by its biological birth, the two being similar yet not parallel. In biological birth, the baby is separated from the mother's body, and once outside, the umbilical cord is cut, leaving the baby to manage its biological functions—breathing, pumping blood, and the like—on its own. This is not to say that the baby is autonomous; quite the contrary. In many respects, it remains dependent on the other, for example, for nourishment and protection from cold or other dangers. Some biological beings are much better equipped at birth in this regard; think of a horse or a whale. Although every birth creates a distance between mother and child, this distance is neither complete nor static but increases as development progresses. The resulting distance is accompanied by a void, immediately experienced by the baby as an unpleasant state to be resolved. This phase is characterized by rapprochement behaviors (Mahler et al., 1975). The young child tolerates a certain distance but becomes fearful when it becomes too overwhelming, prompting an urgent need to alleviate this fear. For instance, when the mother leaves the room and is no longer visible, the baby perceives her absence as her non-existence. When she returns, the baby's joy knows no bounds. This dynamic of disappearance and reappearance marks the beginning of the child's psychic birth. The absence of the mother forces the child to imagine her, to represent her mentally, or even to hallucinate her presence. Yet this is not all; the mental representation of the mother must be complemented by a symbolic representation—technically, the articulation or thought of the absent object. This moment is revolutionary in every person's development and is essential for becoming a fully realized human being. Here too, distance plays a determining and conditional role.

Thus, we can establish that distance is necessary for visual perception and that this also applies to symbolic representation. In both cases, distance emerges as a chasm, corresponding to the gap in being that countless philosophers have discussed and which we recognize as a sine qua non.

These two developmental steps are described by Lacan in the "mirror stage" (Lacan, 1955) and the Law of the Father (Lacan, 1955–1956). During the mirror stage, the child enters the imaginary order, where perception occurs. The introduction of the Law of the Father marks the transition to the symbolic order. In both transitions, a distance from the object is created—first imaginary, then symbolic—leaving a void, a gap in the being of the subject. Lacan entwines the symbolic law with sexuality: "The subject finds its place in a preformed symbolic apparatus that contains the law in sexuality. And this law alone enables the subject to realise his sexuality on the symbolic level" (Lacan, 1955–1956). This human condition is accompanied by the desire to fill this gap. It is on this point that Lacan diverges from Freud, replacing the concept of drive with that of desire.

The young child is not, from the outset, aware of itself, the objects, or the people around it. According to Freud, autoerotic drives initially dominate, with no awareness of the ego and minimal awareness of the external world. A quote clarifies this: "the ego must be developed. The autoerotic drives are original; alongside autoeroticism, a new psychic process must emerge through which narcissism is created." Furthermore: "We assert that man has two primal sexual objects: himself and the nurturing woman, and in doing so, we propose the primary narcissism of every man, which may be expressed as dominant in his choice of object" (Freud, 1914). The question then arises: how does the child develop into a being with a sense of self and awareness of the Other? This begins with the exteriority postulated by Lacan in the mirror stage (Lacan, 1949). Drawing on Wallon's observations, Lacan emphasized the implications of these behaviors for the child's psychological development and their contribution to identity formation.

The behaviors observed during the mirror stage serve as models for all forms of perception—sight, hearing, smell, touch, and taste. Lacan encapsulates this constellation within the concept of the imaginary order. In relation to the psychopathology of perception, which is examined extensively in this book, a deeper exploration of the mirror stage is instructive.

When the child begins to relate the real other to its mirror image, it cannot initially distinguish between the two. For the child, both observations are of equal quality, and it perceives the possibility of being in two places simultaneously. This phenomenon is immediately linked to the doppelgänger experience in Capgras syndrome, discussed in Chapter 8.

When the child hears its name, it turns toward its reflection and extends its arms. Wallon highlights the exteriority of this representation. Upon hearing its name, the child directs its attention to the visual image in the mirror, rather than to its proprioception—its internal bodily awareness. This also enables the child to perceive itself in the mirror as a whole, in contrast to its fragmented perception of its body when looking directly at itself.

The child is confronted with the task of limiting itself to a single location in the room, rather than occupying two simultaneously. This is only possible when perception is detached from reality. Once this revolutionary step is taken, the child realizes that reality is no longer inextricably linked to sensory perception. Sensory impressions thus no longer coincide with reality. From this point on, proprioception assumes primacy. This marks the beginning of the symbolization process. The symbolic function allows the perception of one's own body, the self, to be experienced not as reality but as a sign—one that belongs to the symbolic order.

In describing the mirror stage, the symbolization process also becomes intertwined with the theoretical depiction of the child's development. The question arises as to whether the imaginary process can be strictly separated from the symbolization process, despite their differing orders. In both, distance from reality is fundamental.

Here, nothingness emerges. As we have seen, the child's development entails a dual distancing: one in perception and another in the onset of the symbolization process. This staged distancing occurs during separation—what Lacan terms castration, as it is both painful and irrevocable.

The space created by this double separation contains a void, a nothingness. Through this, the subject begins to differentiate itself from the object with which it initially coincided. This separation occurs in two places: between the subject and the external object, and within the subject itself, creating a separation from its own body. This latter split is termed alienation by Lacan. This internal separation initiates the symbolization process, enabling the subject to signify itself and acquire an identity.

The emergence of nothingness in separation mirrors the fundamental gap between word and object, a theme revisited throughout this book. This gap, this impossibility, arises wherever the symbolic is involved—including in science. I will explore this further in the next chapter.

5

NOTHINGNESS AND SCIENCE

Scientists often feel uncomfortable when confronted with nothingness. This discomfort also applies to the subject, who has found a creative escape through language, only to repeatedly encounter this nothingness again. Scientists seek to objectify this nothingness, but object and subject remain fundamentally opposed, making their integration challenging.

Science aims to understand objects, while the human sciences focus on exploring the subject. Whereas science often claims to have "discovered" the object, the human sciences repeatedly confront the gap between humans and things. Psychiatry, positioned at this intersection, must strive to integrate these two perspectives without falling into reductive determinism.

The practitioners of the positive sciences who study matter in the broadest sense of the term feel uneasy about philosophy, which addresses the status of being and also of nothingness. The natural scientist examines matter: its intrinsic properties and the interrelationships between material entities. Matter adheres to Newton's laws and the theory of relativity, although much remains unknown. However, when confronted with negative matter, of which the black hole is an example, the natural scientist seeks a way to express it in a formula. In doing so, language and mathematics intersect to articulate something in a negative statement. Mathematics employs the "-" sign for this, while language typically uses the word "not" or the prefix "un."

Like all people, the physicist relies on language or mathematics to formulate reality. This necessitates the use of signs and words which, like all symbols, impose a degree of separation from the object.

DOI: 10.4324/9781003675389-8

The question arises whether the same physicist perceives anything when a black hole or negative matter "appears." The absence of perception seems paradoxical. Language and mathematics enable the concept of nothingness. Perception, however, fails us when we "see" nothing. It is precisely thought that permits the possibility of the negative, of absence. Black holes are not directly observed; they are inferred through reasoning and calculations based on the behavior of electromagnetic waves in space. This reasoning or formulation is always mediated by language or its derivatives, such as mathematical calculations.

Science involves observation and interpretation. Early in the last century, Edmund Husserl examined the status of science and expressed profound concern about its trajectory, even referring to a crisis in the sciences (Husserl, 1937). He particularly criticized reductionism, whereby the subjective is subsumed into the doctrine of objectivity as the ideal of science. In this framework, there exists only one truth, which excludes the subject as it is deemed a contaminant of the scientific endeavor. This critique of dominant science was articulated almost a century ago, but it has largely been ignored. It is nevertheless maintained that the subjective transcends the material, that transcendence exists, and in the Anglo-Saxon world, one speaks of "emergence" (Jaegwon Kim, 1993; David Chalmers, 1996). The subject holds a distinct status that is intrinsic to perception. Even the "hard" sciences should acknowledge this.

Can the Gap in Science Be Closed?

Science is preoccupied with the object and claims to have developed methods capable of comprehensively mapping reality. This objectifying approach has achieved much in the natural sciences, yet there always remains an elusive aspect beyond its grasp. Fortunately, scientists have recognized this themselves, notably Werner Heisenberg, who articulated the uncertainty principle in *Physics and Philosophy* (Heisenberg, 1958). This principle, named after him, addresses the subjective dimension inherent in observation. In essence, the subjective element of observation plays a determining role in the perception of any phenomenon. Perception always involves the subject. Machines, such as robots, do not perceive; they merely register. The data collected by computers require interpretation, which involves human consciousness. The unquestioning presentation of statistical figures as truth often neglects the interpretative dimension these data are subject to. How often do we hear that something is "scientifically proven," conferring upon it the status of truth and foreclosing any further discussion?

Science's preoccupation with objectivity has marginalized the subjective. All perception passes through the consciousness of the subject. This is the gap in science, corresponding to Heisenberg's uncertainty principle. One might see this as a deficiency, but it simultaneously opens up possibilities. This subjective gap stimulates thought, discussion, deliberation, and creativity, including imagination and desire. Science benefits from this through the exploration of new frontiers. We engage with reality through words, but words and symbols are not the same as things (Foucault, 1966). The symbolic system of words and signs hovers above reality, occasionally seeming to connect with it, yet always retaining an element of uncertainty.

The question is whether this gap in the objective domain can ever be closed, and whether we should even desire it to be. Philosophically speaking, the gap in being is a sine qua non for consciousness. No, the hole in being cannot be closed, and yes, it is a condition for the existence of consciousness, of which perception is a part.

If science aims to be universal and uphold its claim to truth, it must accommodate the subjective. This is particularly pertinent in psychology. A psychology without a subject is either a false science or not a science at all. Psychology, and psychiatry in its wake, aspires to objectivity, as evidenced by its reliance on statistical data and its mechanical model of human beings. By ignoring the subjective, it risks missing the mark and remaining confined to pure materialism.

Psychoanalysis, too, suffers from a fascination with objective discourse. Trends in neuropsychoanalysis reflect this tendency, as seen in efforts to reduce the unconscious and repression to neuronal functions (cf. Solms, 2021a, 2021b). Psychoanalysis must champion the subjective against the encroachment of objectivism, both through its theoretical framework and its methods of treatment. Sadly, psychoanalysis has nearly disappeared from psychiatry, while psychology students are taught that it has been excluded from the curriculum because it is "unscientific."

Fortunately, there remain psychoanalysts who recognize the existence of a hole in being, located in the unconscious. Besides Lacan, Bion also regarded psychoanalysis as an opportunity to guide the analysand closer to their subjective truth, concealed within the unconscious (Lacan, 1958–1959; Bion, 1965).

6

NOTHINGNESS AS A CREATIVE MOMENT

Despite its challenges, nothingness fosters creativity and desire. This openness to possibilities serves as a vital force for human growth, particularly in the face of existential gaps that arise throughout life.

The impossibility (space) between word and thing is filled with the symbolic of the word and the imaginary of the gaze in an attempt to fill this uncomfortable gab. This gives room for imagination and creativity.

This assertion has been discussed earlier in this book. This underlines that it is not so much a matter of a handicap that the language system that people have in common, but that it provides unprecedented possibilities of freedom and creativity. This has to do with the structure of language, which has an infinite number of possible combinations. It is precisely this symbolic distance from the real that enables man to do something outside the reality of the real that makes that real his own, and as we also know, that does not always benefit us.

The dialectic between word and thing as the most elementary relationship between the Symbolic and the Real has an everlasting character because they are irreducible to each other.

To comprehend the status and origin of nothingness, one can follow the philosophical trajectory established since ancient Greek times. However, it is also both feasible and more pertinent to our subject to explore the birth of the subject itself. This can be approached from a historical perspective or a clinical viewpoint. I opt for the latter, while not hesitating to incorporate historical and philosophical elements wherever relevant.

In Chapter 4, which examined the fundamental impossibilities in thought, the psychological development of the child was discussed. In this

DOI: 10.4324/9781003675389-9

chapter, we focus more closely on what nothingness signifies for the creative capacity of humans in relation to science and culture.

With Lacan, the purely biological is displaced by an interactional and dialectical event. Intentionality and motivation are no longer immanent to matter but instead acquire a transcendental status. Lacan's fundamental stance liberates a purely biological etiology from its physicalist constraints.

The gap in being is not resolved by tautology but is instead filled by something of a different order: the imaginary and the symbolic. This shift naturally provides an entirely different perspective on the mind–body problem that dominates psychiatry and much of philosophy, where reductive approaches have offered constrained solutions. To suggest that this paradigm shift would have no implications for psychiatric practice would, of course, be mistaken.

The concept of a defective subject is also marked by impossibilities. By definition, the subject is a shared subject, a being that, through speech, continuously reiterates the fact that words and things do not coincide. With every spoken word, a hole is created in the subject's being. The next word does the same, and so it continues until death, which ultimately silences this cycle.

This situation may appear disadvantageous, but nothing could be further from the truth. It is precisely this impossibility of aligning word and thing that opens the door to communication, the practice of science, and the creation of poetry. In other words, this gap creates the freedom to imagine and to innovate.

The handicap of being a shared subject also enables (self-)consciousness. One's relationship with one's own body, or oneself, is contingent on language, which is mediated by the symbolic and supported by the imaginary, wherein the senses play a role. Language is necessary to signify oneself. The symbolic is both the cause and effect of the shared subject. Within this framework, Cartesian dualism seems to be revitalized, albeit without reference to a *res cogitans*. The new dualism resides within the split of the subject itself. The subject is divided from a part of its own being and has become estranged from its materiality through the process of symbolization. By entering the symbolic order, the subject distances itself from itself. Lacan describes this as the *sujet barré* (barred subject).

Another difficulty arises concerning the symbolization of the self: the free-floating relationship between word and thing. There is no fixed, one-to-one correspondence between the two. These relationships shift over time, akin to the way air moves across water, constantly altering positions. The interaction between air and water is never static. Similarly, in the language game, the relationship to reality is ever-changing. Yet this variability permits boundless freedom of thought and opens the door to creativity. At the same time, these unlimited possibilities introduce the potential for psychosis. Here, the symbolic assumes a life of its own, disregarding the fixed conventions that enable mutual understanding. For the psychotic, common sense is anything but common. This possibility emerges from the fundamental impossibility between word and thing, as noted earlier. The roots of this disconnection can often, though not always, be traced to an individual's history.

Nothingness thus holds a fundamental status for the subject. It signifies the objects surrounding oneself and the self as an object, enabling a relationship with the Other, as well as the existence of (self-)consciousness.

Nothingness generates desire—a striving to fill the void created by separation. By now, it should be clear that this is unattainable, as signs attempt to fill this void with new symbols, which in turn create yet another gap in the being of things and in the subject itself. Desire endures as long as life persists. It is humanity's destiny to shape its desire, though this is invariably frustrating, as the endpoint is only reached in death.

The actualization of desire manifests in countless forms and is often accompanied by varying experiences of pleasure. Not only do artists use their unique talents to express desire, but less artistically inclined individuals can also employ their creativity to give form to their yearning. The examples are too numerous to count. According to Lacan, speech is the ideal medium for expressing desire, precisely because the object of desire is never fully attained—a condition that would otherwise signify death. Thus, speech becomes the sublime articulation of desire.

Scientists, too, are subject to the dynamics of desire. They seek truth in reality but encounter the same impossibility as every human being. As a result, science, like desire, will never reach an endpoint, for the expression of scientific inquiry can never fully coincide with the reality it seeks to understand.

This also clarifies why science cannot resolve the mind–body problem. Science aspires to objectivity, which necessitates the exclusion of all subjectivity—a fundamentally unachievable goal, both within the natural sciences and the human sciences.

The obsessive pursuit of objectivity has facilitated the deep encroachment of naturalism into the human sciences. Behaviorists are not the only ones influenced by this materialist discourse; even some psychoanalysts are affected. Phenomenologists, for their part, defer the decisive debate about the relationship between mind and body by appealing to their *episteme*[1].

As discussed earlier in Chapter 4 regarding child development, it is worth revisiting the empty space created during the process of castration. The separation between mother and child generates a void, fundamental to the emergence of imagination and symbolization. Imagination and the symbolic are the means by which this empty space is filled. For most individuals, this occurs naturally; for others, the process falters. Some, however, develop exceptional abilities in these areas, as evidenced in artists. Visual artists excel in the domain of the imaginary, while writers and poets cultivate their talents within the symbolic. To become subjects, all individuals must navigate these steps to fill the gap created by separation—a profoundly transformative endeavor that not everyone can achieve.

When this structuring process of separation falters, it can result in severe issues, such as psychosis. In later life, these disruptions leave traces, manifesting as hallucinations in the realm of the imaginary and delusions within the symbolic.

In Part three of this book, we will examine three patients with psychotic experiences to illustrate how a failed structuring of the subject can manifest.

Note

1 Epistème (Gr. ἐπιστημε) is a term from phenomenology that indicates that the judgment (including the diagnosis) about a phenomenon is suspended, postponed in order to give the subjective in the observation the opportunity to process things and attach meaning to them.

PART 3

Three Experiences of Nothingness in the Clinic

Introduction

In the following three chapters, I will delve into the phenomenon of nothingness as observed in clinical settings. These cases involve distinct syndromes: Cotard's syndrome, where patients deny having certain organs such as the heart, lungs, or brain; Capgras syndrome, characterized by a misidentification of the Other, such as perceiving one's mother as someone else; and negative hallucination, which entails the complete erasure of the perception of a person or object. Unlike Capgras syndrome, which involves misrecognition, negative hallucination directly impacts the perceptual experience itself.

In recent years, my clinical work has gravitated toward themes central to child development and their enduring impact on the adult psyche. This exploration has intersected with three intellectual currents: the philosophical concept of nothingness, the clinical experiences of negativity, and the developmental implications of nothingness in childhood. These three threads converge at a singular focus: the concept of nothingness. To elucidate this topic, I will address it from three angles: the clinical perspective, the psychological development of the child, and the philosophical understanding of nothingness.

Clinically, I encountered three patients whose experiences were intimately tied to notions of nothingness or absence. These cases included Cotard's and Capgras syndromes, as well as a patient manifesting negative hallucination.

DOI: 10.4324/9781003675389-10

In the forthcoming chapters, I will examine the clinical manifestations of the negative through these syndromes. All three—Cotard's syndrome, Capgras syndrome, and negative hallucination—are psychotic in nature. Cotard's syndrome involves a psychotic experience of one's own body, characterized by a profound disconnection or denial of its existence. Capgras syndrome represents a psychotic denial of the Other's identity, which can sometimes extend to a denial of the self, as seen in the phenomenon of duplication. Negative hallucination is a psychotic denial of objects, which may include parts of the self, resulting in a profound perceptual absence.

Unlike delusions, which are categorized as thought disorders, negative hallucination is considered a perceptual disturbance. However, negative hallucinations can lead to interpretative distortions that, in some cases, culminate in delusional disorders. These clinical instances reveal the complex interplay between perception, identity, and the profound impact of negation in the human experience.

A book has recently been published entitled Negative Hallucinosis in Wilfred Bion's Theory of Transformations: On Finding One's Ghost (Barahona, 2025), which focuses on Bion's views and compares them with those of Green (1993) and Meltzer and Scolmati (2009). Bion assumes that transformations take place in the field of perception under the influence of severely traumatic events such as he himself experienced during the First World War (Bion, 1965). Transformations in hallucinosis refer to the process by which unprocessed, unrepresentable psychic material (raw emotional experiences) manifests as hallucinations or pseudo-perceptions. These "transformations" occur when the mind fails to engage in meaningful thought processes. For Bion, thinking develops as a capacity to process **β-elements** (raw, unprocessed sensory and emotional experiences) into **α-elements** (thoughts and symbols) through the **α-function.** When this process fails, the psyche resorts to hallucinosis: a mode of perceiving unprocessed material as if it were external reality. Hallucinosis is defensive and regressive, reflecting a failure to symbolize or represent. Lacan's views on psychosis differ from those of Bion. Lacan emphasizes the failure of the symbolic through the foreclosure/rejection of the Name-of-the-Father. The psychotic subject has no or an inadequate defense against the Real, which overwhelms him. In Bion, perception is paramount, which includes emotions in Lacan's view. Emotions belong to the order of the Imaginary. Bion believes that in psychosis, both the positive and the negative hallucination are the result of a transformation of perception.involves an inability to differentiate internal from external reality. According to Lacan the defense against the Real is of the symbolic order. In this, the structuring capacity of language plays a fundamental role. In Bion, hallucinosis is a phenomenon that occurs within the field of perception, the imaginary order. Whether thinking, which is in fact a speech act, also plays a role in this is not so clear in Bion.

Despite the differences between Lacan and Bion, both concepts grapple with absences—whether of perception (negative hallucinosis) or of being (nothingness). They also share a preoccupation with the limits of human experience and representation, making them relevant in discussions of trauma, creativity, and existential anxiety.

Barahona's work bridges these ideas by showing how negative hallucinosis interacts with the voids of the mind, contributing to a psychoanalytic understanding of nothingness (Barahona, 2025). This connection enriches the clinical and philosophical discourse, linking the unrepresented (negative hallucinosis) with broader existential gaps (nothingness).

Here are the three clinical vignettes that have a negative signature of reality interpretation.

7

AS IN A BLACK MIRROR

Cotard's Syndrome

This chapter delves into Cotard's syndrome, a rare and complex psychiatric condition characterized by delusions of non-existence or profound nihilism. The patient's experience of nothingness is marked by an extreme form of detachment, where even the body is perceived as void. These perceptions illustrate the intricate interplay between the Real, Imaginary, and Symbolic dimensions, offering valuable insights into the psychotic experience.

For me, the most compelling manifestation of nothingness is the experience of not existing. According to many psychiatrists, this phenomenon falls under Cotard's syndrome, typically involving the absence of a vital organ such as the heart, brain, or lungs. The case described here, however, concerns a woman who not only ignores her identity but also denies her physical presence entirely. Despite this profound detachment, she retains a sense of humor and demonstrates an ability to empathize with others. For instance, she acknowledges that I, as her therapist, can see and hear her speak, yet she maintains that she does not exist. This manifestation of "being nothing" represents a far-reaching error of interpretation, surpassing the notion of merely feeling worthless.

Le délire de négation, or nihilistic delusion, continues to present significant challenges for psychiatry. In practice, encountering a patient who asserts that they are dead triggers a near-irresistible urge to refute or contradict the claim. After overcoming the initial bewilderment that such a meeting provokes, one begins to grapple with the question of how such a "nothing" thought could have taken root in the patient's mind.

DOI: 10.4324/9781003675389-11

I recall my first encounter with a patient suffering from Cotard's syndrome some 30 years ago. She entered my consulting room and asked me to prepare a death certificate for her. Stunned, I failed to document a single detail from our meeting. During the session, I encouraged her to continue the conversation, hoping to understand her better before making any conclusions. She resisted, insisting that her death was obvious and that issuing a death certificate was a mere administrative task. After our second meeting, she disappeared, and I never saw her again. Her absence was as enigmatic as her condition, and I was left pondering her fate, still shaken by the encounter.

More recently, I met a second patient with Cotard's syndrome, this time within a clinical setting. The nursing staff had informed me that she urgently wished to see a doctor. Our initial meeting was as shocking as the one decades prior. "Doctor, will you cut my head off?" she asked. Despite my many years in psychiatry, this request was profoundly unsettling—certainly not an everyday occurrence. It was significant enough to share with colleagues.

This patient had spent years in a psychiatric hospital. Her husband visited her twice a week and, in the interim, had formed a new relationship with another partner—a development she was aware of and approved, as she believed herself to be dead. Her conviction of non-existence shaped her reality. In this chapter, I recount her story, juxtaposing her phenomenal world with that of contemporary psychiatric science. Her voice will be heard throughout, revealing how her words and perspectives often left others astounded. Her undeniable sense of humor will also emerge, providing a glimpse into her unique, albeit tragic, worldview.

But let's start with the science that doesn't quite know how to deal with the phenomenon of a paradoxical contradiction that this patient presents to us like a sphinx with statements such as: "I'm dead" and "End my life."

In this case, the relationship with the Other[1] is central, in which both Symbolic and Imaginary elements are discussed. In general, the subject is subjected to the Other. That is to say, the young child first mirrors itself to the Other, who is usually represented by the mother and father, and then starts speaking, adopting the language that also comes from the Other. Both events, the Imaginary of mirroring and the Symbolic of speaking, involve an identification with something that comes from outside. That is why in this case one speaks of *extimacy* as opposed to intimacy. The transfer of the Other always takes place through real persons who are carriers of the culture in which a child ends up.

Through alienation, the split in the subject between the being of the Real and the Symbolic of language creates a caesura in the self, through which the individual is given the opportunity to speak and thus becomes part of the symbolic world of culture. According to Lacan, the subject is the effect of speech. In a self-reflecting position, the subject distances itself from itself, initially in an Imaginary way and then in a Symbolic sense. The self is desubstantiated and incorporated into the Symbolic order. Then the subject is in a position to signify itself and to provide itself with an identity, to provide itself with a sign.

In psychosis, something goes wrong in this symbolization process. The symbolization takes a false route in which a *fausse route* of word and thing can occur. From the symbolic position, the subject can think of anything, the strangest situations, and also completely impossible ones. Because we usually think the same things as our neighbors in the face of reality, we are not considered crazy and think we are quite normal. This common sense is often hard to find in psychotics. Then they think, for example, that they can fly or that they are the president of America. It can even go so far that they experience themselves as non-existent, as is the case with Cotard's syndrome.

This absurd inconsistency makes us think. How is it possible that you can ignore an obvious experience, even think it away, delete it from consciousness? That is the question we must ask ourselves, also in modern psychiatry. Attributing this phenomenon to a defect in the brain seems to me as absurd as the phenomenon itself.

Cotard and the Nihilistic Delusion

It is probable that Jules Cotard was the first to publish about negative hallucinations, and it concerned a patient who thought she was dead (Cotard, 1884). The name of Hippolyte Bernheim is also mistakenly mentioned, but his publication on the same phenomenon is of a later date, 1888 (Blom, 2010). A variant of this remarkable phenomenon is the belief that one does not have a heart or brain, about which I have published together with Thierry Verplancke (de Kroon & Verplancke, 2017). Not long after Cotard's publication, Freud mentioned the negative hallucination in *Psychic Treatment (Treatment of the Soul)* (Freud, 1890). Since then, he has regularly referred to this phenomenon.

It is not so surprising that Freud was familiar with this phenomenon because from October 1885 to February 1886, he stayed as an assistant physician in the Salpêtrière in Paris, where Jules Martin Charcot held sway and counted Jules Cotard among his students. Freud must have been struck by the existence of the negative hallucination, given the many times he returns to it in his texts and that this phenomenon has even given a twist to his conceptions of perception. I will come back to that later.

The medical history that Freud published together with Joseph Breuer concerned the story of Miss Anna O. During the treatment, Freud noticed that her condition was worsening, so he called a colleague for a consultation. Anna O. repeatedly failed to notice this colleague. She simply didn't see him while he was in the room. Only when the doctor, irritated, blew smoke in her face did she become aware of the strange doctor, flee to the door, and fall unconscious to the floor (Breuer & Freud, 1893).

Another negative hallucination is described in the history of the Wolfman. At the age of four and a half, the patient experienced something strange while playing in the garden with his *njanja* (nanny). He was carving the bark of an oak tree with a knife, the same oak tree from his dream with the seven wolves. Suddenly, he noticed that he had cut off his little finger, although it was still attached by a thin piece of skin. He became anxious but felt no pain. He quickly sat down on the couch next to his *njanja* without saying anything. A moment later, he dared to look at his hand and saw that his little finger was intact again. Freud called this a negative hallucination and associated it with the castration fear that played a central role in the history of the Wolfman (Freud, 1919).

A few years earlier, Freud had written a more theoretical text, *Metapsychological Supplement to the Theory of Dreams* (Freud, 1914). In this work, he compared hallucinations with dreams. Freud distinguished between the primary process and the secondary process, where the dream belongs to the first and reality testing occurs in the second. The dream image persists but gains meaning only through processing in the secondary process. Freud pointed out for the first time that both dreams and hallucinations stem from primary (primitive) narcissism. However, in hallucinations, the reality check disappears, whereas the dreamer knows upon waking that it was a dream.

André Green devoted a chapter to the negative hallucination in his *Le travail du négatif*. He revisited Freud's *Metapsychological Supplement* and noted that Freud's view marked a radical shift in his theory of hallucinations. Freud transitioned his focus from the opposition between perception and memory to the representation within the subject, where no difference exists between a dream image and a hallucination. Initially, the emphasis was on the object perceived by the subject, but it now shifted to the subject itself and the process of perception. Green stressed the revolutionary significance of Freud's insights on negative hallucination, which involve the denial of unpleasant experiences (Green, 1993).

To my knowledge, Lacan never explicitly spoke of negative hallucination, but the concept of negativity or nothingness holds a prominent place in his theory. As mentioned earlier, the separation of the subject creates a void—a nothingness—that demands to be filled. This void is filled by the *objet petit a*, which primarily has an Imaginary character and is inherently tied to perception and interpretation.

In contemporary psychoanalytic texts, negative hallucinations are often explained as a regression comparable to preconscious perceptions or infantile amnesia (Brakel, 1989; Hazif-Thomas et al., 2014; Hazif-Thomas et al., 2016).

Negative Hallucinations and Cotard's Syndrome

The question remains whether Cotard's syndrome involves a negative hallucination. If someone believes they have no organs, we are clearly dealing with a delusional disorder. Knowledge of the body's interior—such as the heart or liver—comes from science and education, part of the Symbolic order, not merely the Imaginary. If you are alive and healthy, you are unaware of your organs, which is why you cannot normally believe you lack them, unlike the hypochondriac delusion.

Clérambault associated negative hallucinations with automatisms of thought (Clérambault, 1942). He viewed hallucinations, which classical psychiatry considered perceptual disorders, as thought disorders and thus part of the Symbolic order.

In the time of Jules Cotard in the late 19th century, psychiatry was dominated by naturalism. Although Charcot could distinguish epilepsy from conversion symptoms, he remained convinced that hysteria had an organic basis. Similarly, Cotard believed that delusions, including the nihilistic delusion, had an organic substrate.[2]

To this day, naturalism remains dominant in psychiatry and neurology, attributing psychoses to brain defects. Despite its shortcomings, this perspective has persisted unchallenged in mainstream psychiatry.

The nihilistic delusion represents a profound misinterpretation of one's own body, with far-reaching consequences for perception that may lead to negative hallucinations. Generally, the intellectual abilities of patients with Cotard's syndrome remain intact. They can perform the tasks required for daily life, yet their conviction that they are dead can render them completely incapacitated.

What does this case teach us? It demonstrates that the three orders of the Real, the Symbolic, and the Imaginary are inseparably intertwined and cannot be reduced to one another. They are held together by a certain law or symptom that "afflicts" every subject. Simply diminishing symptoms, as is often done in contemporary psychiatric practice, can have disastrous consequences, as it disrupts a certain balance within the subject (cf. Prigogine & Stengers, 1985).

As humans are speaking beings, the Symbolic order exerts the greatest influence on experience. The interpretation of reality—the act of giving meaning to what is observed—defines the Other-truth level for the subject.

This subjective interpretation often differs from the perceptions of others or the common sense shared within a society. For the psychotic subject, the Symbolic has run amok, detached from its anchors in the Real. The psychotic subject becomes disconnected from the Other and follows their own course.

Clinical experience confirms that psychosis does not always manifest itself overtly; in some cases, it only disturbs certain aspects of perception or interpretation. This aligns with the isolation of the psychotic within their own world, which classical psychiatry once described as an autistic feature of psychosis.

Psychiatric research and treatment must devote greater attention to the Symbolic dimension of human existence rather than focusing exclusively on the brain, where—according to some—nothing is found that pertains to the Symbolic. The Symbolic is, at most, an effect of the complex interplay between the subject and the Other. Neuroscientific findings themselves fall under the regime of the Symbolic, as they must be interpreted to gain meaning.

Thus, the psychiatric paradigm could shift toward a subject-centered approach that acknowledges the intertwining of the Real, the Symbolic, and the Imaginary. These three orders are irreducible to one another, a fact that bears repeating. However, the Symbolic order remains paramount: without the Symbolic—language, naming—we cannot even represent the Real or the Imaginary.

In summary, Cotard's syndrome and nihilistic delusions exemplify the limits of a naturalistic understanding of psychiatry. The phenomenon reveals the failure of reductionist approaches that attempt to locate the origins of psychosis solely within the biological domain. At the same time, it highlights the importance of the Symbolic order, the realm of language, meaning, and interpretation, in shaping human experience.

By examining Cotard's syndrome through this lens, we gain insight into the profound complexity of psychotic phenomena. The Symbolic dimension allows us to move beyond the purely organic to consider the psychic and relational aspects of the subject. Only then can we do justice to the intricate interplay between body, mind, and culture—a relationship that continues to elude simplistic, naturalistic explanations.

The Symbolic and Its Role in Psychosis

The phenomenon of nihilistic delusions, as seen in Cotard's syndrome, underscores the inherent limitations of a strictly biological approach to psychiatry. While the brain and its functions are undoubtedly important, the reduction of complex psychotic phenomena to mere neuronal activity overlooks the fundamental role of the Symbolic order. This order—comprising language, culture, and meaning—is central to human existence and identity.

Lacan's theory reminds us that the subject is born into language, which comes from the Other. It is through the Symbolic that we interpret reality, give meaning to our experiences, and construct our identities. This process involves alienation because the subject adopts a language that originates outside of themselves. The very act of speaking requires a split in the subject—a caesura between the Real and the Symbolic—through which the subject becomes a participant in the symbolic world.

However, in psychosis, something goes awry in this process of symbolization. Lacan describes psychosis as resulting from the *foreclosure of the Name-of-the-Father* (forclusion du Nom-du-Père). This foreclosure prevents the anchoring of the Symbolic within the Real, creating a gap where meaning fails to stabilize. The psychotic subject is left adrift, unable to construct a coherent interpretation of reality. Instead, they develop delusions, hallucinations, or other distorted perceptions to fill this void.

In the case of Cotard's syndrome, the subject's nihilistic delusion—that they do not exist or lack vital organs—reveals the breakdown of the Symbolic order. Their experience of nothingness is not a simple denial of existence but rather a radical failure of symbolization. The void that arises is filled not with the stabilizing *objet petit a*, as Lacan might describe, but with a paradoxical conviction of emptiness. This "nothingness" becomes the subject's reality, one that cannot be corrected by appealing to common sense or the Real.

Scotomization and the Role of the Imaginary

The French concept of *scotomization*—the selective "disappearance" of reality—provides another lens through which to understand Cotard's syndrome. Scotomization refers to the obstruction or distortion of perception, where certain elements of reality become obscured or erased. In Cotard's syndrome, this manifests as the belief that vital organs are absent, or that the self no longer exists.

This phenomenon parallels Lacan's *mirror stage*, in which the Imaginary plays a crucial role in shaping the subject's identity. During this stage, the child sees its reflection in the mirror and identifies with this external image—a process that establishes the *ideal ego*. However, in psychosis, the Imaginary fails to support the subject's coherence, and the reflection of the self becomes distorted or absent altogether. The result is a fractured identity, where the subject cannot reconcile their existence with their perception of reality.

A Call for a Paradigm Shift in Psychiatry

The persistence of naturalistic explanations within contemporary psychiatry reflects a blind spot in our understanding of psychosis. While advances in neuroscience have provided valuable insights into the brain's role in mental illness, they have done little to illuminate the subjective experience of the psychotic patient. The nihilistic delusion challenges us to move beyond reductionist approaches and engage with the Symbolic and Imaginary dimensions of human experience.

To address the complexity of psychosis, psychiatry must adopt a more holistic framework that integrates the Real, the Symbolic, and the Imaginary. This framework acknowledges that the subject cannot be reduced to their biology alone but must be understood in relation to language, culture, and the Other.

The nihilistic delusion reveals the fragility of the Symbolic order and the profound consequences of its collapse. It reminds us that the subject's experience of reality is shaped not only by the brain but also by the intricate interplay of meaning, perception, and identity. By embracing this understanding, psychiatry can better serve the needs of psychotic patients and move closer to a more comprehensive and humane approach to mental illness.

The Limits of the Biological Reduction

Psychiatry's reliance on the biological framework to explain psychotic phenomena often leaves the subjective experience of the patient unaddressed. While the brain can be examined, measured, and mapped, the Symbolic and Imaginary dimensions remain intangible and elusive to purely scientific methods. The nihilistic delusion exemplifies this limitation: it cannot be reduced to a malfunction in brain structure or chemistry alone, as it reflects a collapse of meaning—a failure of symbolization that no brain scan can capture.

The phenomenon of *nothingness*, central to Cotard's syndrome, exposes the gap between body and mind, and between word and thing, that has long troubled philosophy and psychiatry alike. In Lacan's terms, the Symbolic order mediates this gap through language, allowing the subject to articulate their experiences and make sense of their existence. When the Symbolic fails, the Real emerges unmediated, confronting the subject with an overwhelming void. The psychotic delusion is an attempt to bridge this void, to impose meaning on an otherwise incomprehensible experience.

The reductionist approach, which attributes psychotic phenomena to brain defects, overlooks this essential aspect of the subject's experience. Such an approach dismisses the complexity of the human condition, which cannot be understood without considering the interplay between biology, language, and culture. The nihilistic delusion, as seen in Cotard's syndrome, challenges us to recognize the limits of naturalism and to adopt a more inclusive understanding of psychosis.

Subjectivity and the Role of the Other

As humans, we are inherently relational beings. Our sense of self and reality is shaped through our interactions with the Other—the people and cultural structures that surround us. In Cotard's syndrome, the subject's relationship to the Other is profoundly disrupted. The Symbolic fails to anchor their experience of reality, and the Imaginary no longer provides a coherent reflection of the self. The result is an extreme alienation, where the subject denies not only their identity but also their very existence.

In clinical practice, this presents a significant challenge. The therapist or psychiatrist, as the representative of the Other, becomes entangled in the patient's delusion. Attempts to argue against the patient's beliefs—such as proving that they are alive—are futile because the delusion exists outside the framework of common sense. Instead, the therapist must engage with the patient on their own terms, exploring the meaning of their experience without imposing external interpretations.

This requires a shift in psychiatric practice toward a subject-centered approach. By recognizing the importance of language, meaning, and the patient's relationship to the Other, clinicians can better understand the subjective reality of psychotic patients. This approach does not dismiss the biological aspects of mental illness but situates them within the broader context of the subject's lived experience.

The Complexity of the Symbolic, Real, and Imaginary

The intertwining of the Symbolic, Real, and Imaginary is fundamental to understanding Cotard's syndrome and other psychotic phenomena. These three orders, as described by Lacan, cannot be reduced to one another, yet they interact in complex ways to shape the subject's experience of reality.

- *The Symbolic* represents language, meaning, and the structures through which we interpret reality. It provides the framework that allows the subject to signify their experiences and construct an identity.
- *The Imaginary* involves perception, images, and the reflections through which the subject identifies with themselves and the world. It plays a crucial role in forming the subject's ego and sense of self.
- *The Real* refers to what exists beyond language and representation. It is the unmediated, raw experience of reality that cannot be symbolized or integrated into the subject's understanding.

In Cotard's syndrome, the failure of the Symbolic disrupts the subject's relationship to the Imaginary and exposes them to the overwhelming void of the Real. The delusion—that they are dead, or that their organs are missing—reflects an attempt to impose meaning on this void. Yet this meaning is inherently paradoxical, as it denies the very existence of the subject.

Implications for Modern Psychiatry

The study of nihilistic delusions, and Cotard's syndrome in particular, highlights the need for a more nuanced approach to psychiatry—one that transcends the limitations of naturalism and embraces the complexity of human experience. While neuroscience and biological psychiatry have made significant advances, they cannot fully account for the subjective realities of psychotic patients.

Psychiatry must recognize that the human subject is not merely a biological organism but a being embedded in language, culture, and relationships. The Symbolic, Imaginary, and Real are not peripheral to the study of mental illness; they are central to understanding the subject's experience and the nature of psychotic phenomena.

By integrating these dimensions into psychiatric practice, clinicians can better engage with their patients and address the underlying disruptions that give rise to delusions and other psychotic symptoms. This approach does not reject the biological basis of mental illness but situates it within a broader, more holistic understanding of the human condition.

Conclusion

Cotard's syndrome and the nihilistic delusion force us to confront the limits of our understanding of psychosis. They reveal the fragility of the Symbolic order and the devastating consequences of its collapse. At the same time, they challenge psychiatry to move beyond reductionist approaches and engage with the subjective experience of the psychotic subject.

The integration of the Real, Symbolic, and Imaginary provides a framework for understanding the complexity of psychosis and the interplay of biological, linguistic, and cultural factors. By adopting a subject-centered approach, psychiatry can better serve its patients and address the profound disruptions that lie at the heart of psychotic phenomena.

Cotard's syndrome teaches us that nothingness is not merely an absence but a presence—a void that demands to be filled. It is through the Symbolic that we confront this void and give meaning to our existence. When this process fails, as it does in psychosis, the subject is left to navigate a world where meaning has collapsed, and the Real emerges in its raw, unmediated form.

Notes

1 The Other stands for the entire cultural constellation. The language that carries culture has existed long before we were born. We come, as it were, in a pre-existing situation. It is the others who lead us into the realm of language. Usually these are our parents, extended family, teachers and playmates. They are part of the culture to which the child will belong. Lacan calls this symbolic environment the Other. Without the Other, we as a newborn individual will not speak.

2 This organic naturalistic view was very widespread in medical circles of the time. Freud too stubbornly clung to this, even for the neuroses he was most concerned with. This does not alter the fact that he has discovered and described very subtle psychological patterns. He himself has admitted that the substrate for psychic mechanisms have never been demonstrated by him and others. Good thing, too.

8

THE STRANGER IN OURSELVES

Capgras Syndrome

Capgras Syndrome provides another vivid example of the experience of nothingness in psychosis. Patients believe that their close relations have been replaced by impostors, exposing a fracture in their perception of reality. This phenomenon reflects a breakdown in the symbolic order, leaving the patient stranded in the Imaginary, unable to bridge the gap with the Real.

In the DSM ideology, Capgras syndrome, along with Cotard, Frégoli, and de Clérambault syndromes, is classified as a neurological phenomenon with no identified somatic substrate. We regard all four of these clinical phenomena as disorders of interpretation.

In Capgras syndrome, defense and projection are at work. The patient's true motive is not tolerated—specifically, their defense against feelings of hatred toward their partner, which conflict with the expected positive feelings. It is not so much a matter of repressing negative feelings as creating an empty space where no feelings exist. The interaction between both partners reflects the fact that the partner is neither recognized nor known by the patient.

A 27-year-old woman had recently left her boyfriend. They had moved into a new rental home just days earlier so she could be closer to her work. The abrupt separation was not entirely unexpected for her boyfriend. For years, there had been considerable friction, and they no longer slept together. She often made strange statements that he could not understand. One day she mistook him for a stranger who merely looked like him but was not him—a doppelganger: "You are not John. You are someone else." When she accused him of trying to poison her, it became clear to him that she required psychiatric help. She vehemently disagreed.

DOI: 10.4324/9781003675389-12

After some time, she was persuaded to seek help, not because she thought her beliefs were flawed but because she felt inexplicably exhausted, which had prevented her from working as a nurse for over a year. Through her GP, she was referred to a primary care psychologist, with whom she established a good rapport. However, her complaints of fatigue and gloom deepened, driving her to desperation and thoughts of death. At that time, she fled to her parents, staying with them for three months. When she began suspecting her mother of poisoning her food, the household tension became unbearable. She planned to take her own life.

She visited a local hardware store, purchased a luggage strap and a bag of cement, and hurried to a bridge spanning a wide, deep body of water. She fastened the strap around herself and the cement bag, preparing to jump from the bridge. Fortunately, bystanders intervened, and she was transported by ambulance to our hospital, where she was admitted to the high-intensity care (HIC) department. There, she withdrew into a state of permanent silence. When pressed, she claimed we already knew everything because she had shared it with other care providers.

It emerged that she had previously been admitted to the neighboring PAAZ (Psychiatric Department of a General Hospital), where a psychiatrist diagnosed her with Capgras syndrome. This was based on her misidentification of her boyfriend as a doppelganger and her assertion that her father was not her biological father but also an impostor.

In psychiatry, and even more so in neurology, there is a pronounced tendency to view Delusional Misidentification Syndromes (DMS)—such as Capgras, Cotard, Fregoli, and de Clérambault syndromes—as neurological disorders (Atta, 2006; Anderson, 2016). However, less reductionist perspectives, like that of Salvatore and colleagues, offer a more nuanced understanding. They wrote a well-supported article concluding: "Capgras syndrome was prevalent across a broad spectrum of first-episode psychotic disorders, most often in acute psychoses or with rapid onset" (Salvatore, 2014, p. 261). Their research revealed that Capgras syndrome occurred in 50% of cases of schizophreniform disorders.

Other articles also challenge this biological reductionism, such as Christodoulou's (2018) work, which concludes: "Speculating on these syndromes is a fascinating journey in psychopathology, but although in most cases an organic contributor is present, the great diversity of conditions in which DMSs occur renders the possibility of a unifying hypothesis unlikely" (p. 16).

The myth of Procrustes is often invoked in this context. This figure from mythology invited travelers to stay with him but only had one size bed. Guests who did not fit were either stretched or had their legs shortened to conform. Similarly, patients with Capgras syndrome can be forced into the Procrustean bed of biological reductionism.

Christodoulou and colleagues discovered that Capgras syndrome appears in 26.4% of cases involving dementia and other organic disorders. Additionally, among psychiatric inpatients, 3.11% are reported to have Capgras syndrome. In 92.3% of these cases, the patients are diagnosed with (paranoid) schizophrenia, while 7.69% involve affective disorders (Joseph, 1994).

De Jonghe and Markx attempted to classify and distinguish between pathological and normal misidentification without offering an explanation (de Jonghe and Markx, 1979a). In a subsequent article, they described Capgras syndrome as a pathological phenomenon of negative misidentification rooted in misconception rather than misperception (de Jonghe and Markx, 1979b).

Problem

When confronted with cases like Caroline's, and as with Cotard's syndrome, we initially overcome our astonishment before questioning how it is possible for factual interpretation to deviate so drastically that obvious realities are completely misconstrued. What are the grounds and mechanisms for this derailment? While abnormal neuronal firing or altered pathways in the brain's neuronal network might be suggested, such explanations say little about the root cause of the derailment. A psychologically significant event could potentially initiate a new pathway in the brain, leading to lasting changes over time.

This raises questions about whether the original causality lies in the brain or the environment. If a traumatic event triggers an initial pathway in the neuronal network, how does this lead to an interpretation so far removed from consensus? Was the event severe? Repeated? The answers remain elusive. Practitioners, too, interpret phenomena differently.

Expressing misinterpretation in psychosis through psychological terms has a long history in psychiatry (Freud, 1911; Jackson, 1884; Ey, 1938; Berrios, 1996). However, such interpretations often rely on models developed for psychopathological structures other than psychosis. Freud, for instance, attributed psychosis to the repression of homosexuality (Freud, 1911, 1922). Jackson connected psychosis to evolutionary and dissolutive processes in the central nervous system, a notion later refined by Ey in his organo-dynamism theory (Jackson, 1884; Ey, 1938).

Although these are sophisticated models, they treat the psyche as an epiphenomenon of physical processes rather than a distinct category. This chapter argues for considering the psyche as a separate category, irreducible to the organic without dire consequences. A comprehensive understanding must account for the interplay between physical processes and psychological mechanisms. One cannot exist without the other.

When investigating causes, it is necessary to examine both life events and the symbolic-biological structure intrinsic to human beings. Only the combination of biological and symbolic dimensions provides an adequate explanation. Reducing one to the other constitutes a categorical error. Figures like Damasio and Kandel, who reduce psychological phenomena to biology, fall into this trap (Damasio, 1994; Kandel, 2018).

Biological models leave unresolved issues, such as psychogenesis, the influence of environmental factors, and the origins of consciousness. The mind–body problem persists. Nonetheless, hypotheses offering a more comprehensive view than reductionist biology do exist.

Freud and Lacan on the Doppelganger

Freud linked the double to narcissism and the fear of death (Freud, 1919). Narcissism allows the subject to see themselves as an object of love. In primary narcissism, this is hypothetical; after engaging in object relationships, secondary narcissism emerges. Here, the ego may split, creating an external ego. Freud's ideas resonate with Otto Rank, who described the doppelganger as a charm against death (Rank, 1914).

The splitting of the ego allows the self to experience itself as an object, fostering differentiation and conscience formation. Pathologically, the split-off ego may become autonomous, taking on a chasing role or being idealized. This pattern appears in our patient, who idealizes her alter ego while the "reprehensible" parts remain attached to her self, which she seeks to destroy.

Lacan expanded on this theme in his concept of the Imaginary and the mirror stage (Lacan, 1949, 1966). Between 6 and 18 months, the child identifies with its reflection, forming the ego through identification. This external image brings both joy and alienation, introducing rivalry and aggression.

In this patient's case, developmental disruptions align with Freud's notion of ego splitting and Lacan's ideas on faulty symbolization. Lacan attributes psychosis to the rejection of the "Name-of-the-Father" (Forclusion du Nom-du-Père), impairing the paternal function and Symbolic order. False perceptions arise in the Real, creating fixation on the Imaginary.

Conclusion

Lacan has taken up the theme of the doppelgänger in his development of the Imaginary beginning with the introduction of the mirror stage (Lacan, 1949, 1966). This is the stage in the child's development between 6 and 18 months. The mirror stage describes the formation of the I along the way of identification. The ego is the result of identification with one's own reflection. This is accompanied by an extreme joy ("jubilation"). The mirror image comes from the outside and not from the inside. Before that, the child still experienced itself as a fragmented body ("corps morcelé"). After the mirror stage, the child sees itself as a whole. This transition from fragmented to whole also has a dark side; With the identification with the image outside himself, the child also distances himself from himself, distance from his own origin. With the mirror stage, the child enters into the imaginary order. In Lacan too, the mirror stage and the imaginary order are associated with narcissism. Narcissism is accompanied by rivalry with oneself. The mirror image is there outside the self which gives rise to alienation and aggression.

In the patient described here there is a hiccup in her development that can be traced in the relevant texts of Freud as well as those of Lacan. Freud speaks of a splitting of the ego which, in normal development, gives rise to the formation of conscience. In a pathological development, the split-off ego takes on a life of its own and becomes an institution that must be destroyed. Another possibility is that the unintegrated part is projected outward into a chaser. The next step is that this pursuer is transformed into a doppelganger. There is also a split there.

In Lacan's psychosis, there is a malfunctioning Oedipus complex because the Law-of-the-Father is rejected (*Forclusion du-Nom-du-Père*). As a result, a defect has occurred in the paternal function whereby the symbolic does not function properly. The paternal function is reduced to the imaginary with which the subject gets stuck in the mirror stage where there are doublings that are not symbolized. The false perceptions take place in the Real. The "rejection of the Name-of-the-Father" gives rise to a fixation on the Imaginary and a dysfunctional Symbolic order. In fact, both aspects of this form of psychosis (Capgras syndrome) are manifestations of one and the same mechanism; a different structuring of the subject than is the case with the neurotic.

In a therapeutic sense, there is little one can do but be there for the patient and listen to his story. In this patient's case, it seems that connecting with her quest within the imaginary field is a meaningful therapeutic endeavor. This is apparent from her great interest and activity in art therapy. There she finds her expression.

In this text an attempt has been made to relate the theme of doubling, which is an aspect of Capgras syndrome, with the splitting of the ego that Freud speaks of and the doubling that Lacan talks about in his theory of the mirror stage. Moreover, Lacan makes it clear to us that the stagnant transition from the imaginary, of which the mirror stage is a part, to the symbolic plays a role in the misinterpretation that occurs in the phenomenon of the double. With regard to psychosis, Lacan has taken up Freud's thread about the splitting of the ego and has supplemented it with a theory about defective symbolization. In this text, attention has been paid to both aspects in relation to Capgras syndrome.

Capgras syndrome challenges psychiatry by exposing the intricate interplay between psychological, biological, and symbolic processes. By examining the structural and developmental aspects of misidentification, this chapter highlights the limitations of reductionist approaches and underscores the importance of an integrative framework for understanding psychosis.

9

THE EXPERIENCE OF NOTHINGNESS

In this chapter, a clinical vignette illustrates a patient's subjective encounter with nothingness. This case highlights how the absence of symbolic integration can lead to profound existential crises, showcasing the therapeutic potential of addressing such voids through dialogue and structuralist principles.

The first few times I spoke to Melanie, I found her quite charming. She had a trendy outfit and an engaging way of speaking. To her, there was nothing much wrong, and she found it strange that she had to be admitted with a Judicial Authorization. In her neighborhood, however, she had caused considerable nuisance to the local residents, particularly by collecting waste that she stored in her house. Her nocturnal activities, accompanied by excessively loud music, greatly irritated her neighbors. The rooms of her house were crammed to the ceiling with items she had found on the streets and in rubbish bins. According to the FACT team, staying in her home was no longer safe, neither for herself nor for her environment, particularly regarding hygiene. She used drugs that were sourced for her by "friends." She had started three university degrees but had not completed any of them, one being medicine at the same university where I studied, which created a certain bond between us. She had been in a relationship and had two children, who had been placed in foster care, with whom she had little to no contact.

In the clinic, she was initially placed in the Dual Diagnosis ward to address her addiction. It required significant effort to get to grips with her drug use. She vehemently denied using drugs and offered various medical explanations for why her blood tests might be unreliable. When it was

DOI: 10.4324/9781003675389-13

established that she was using GHB, she was transferred to the psychosis treatment ward. There, she continued her hoarding activities and ensured that "friends" visited her, bringing drugs. During this period, I witnessed her fall into a deep coma three times due to GHB use, each time endangering her life. These events were both tense and deeply impactful for the team. Afterward, Melanie denied everything that had happened—denying any drug use or memory of being unconscious. She did not seem to be lying or repressing the events; for her, they simply did not exist. She could not comprehend our concerns.

At first glance, this behavior might be interpreted as denial or trivialization of the problem, behaviors often seen in addicts. However, she did not give us that impression. Instead, it seemed to be a gap in her existence, something completely non-existent to her.

A clinician might argue against the presence of a negative hallucination, suggesting that drugs—especially GHB—are associated with memory loss. This could indeed have been the case for Melanie, but the counterargument is that her memory function was otherwise intact. Other practitioners and nurses were equally struck by her "denial" of reality, which differed from their experiences with other GHB users. Melanie made an authentic impression on me.

The Negative Hallucination and Nothingness

A negative hallucination revolves around nothingness. The psychotic individual confronted with this phenomenon does not perceive what is undeniably present. This is difficult to articulate, as it goes beyond conventional perception. It is not uncommon for us to overlook something until someone points it out. For instance, you might look at a tree and think you see everything there is to observe: the shape and colors of the branches and leaves, the thickness of the trunk, the height of the tree, and even the blue sky visible through the canopy. Then your companion says, "Do you see those birds on that branch?" You reply, "No, where?" After some guidance, you finally notice two birds perched on a branch. Without your companion's help, you would not have seen them.

However, this is not a negative hallucination. After a corrective prompt, you are able to observe what is there. In a negative hallucination, such correction is futile. The gap in perception persists; something is entirely absent from the picture or sound. When it involves one's own body, the phenomenon moves closer to an unmistakably flawed interpretation. For example, someone denying the presence of their heart, even while standing in front of you, illustrates a different kind of logic. Language plays a crucial role here.

Negative hallucinations often result in part of reality being erased, a process referred to as scotomization, discussed earlier in this text. When the experience of nothingness becomes total and overwhelming, fear arises, which seems incompatible with life. This will be revisited at the conclusion of this text.

Clinical Observations

As with the previous text on Capgras syndrome, it must be noted that phenomena associated with absence are rarely encountered in the clinic. In Capgras syndrome, this absence pertains to identity; in Cotard's syndrome, it involves the conviction of lacking vital organs or even life itself. Here, we are discussing a phenomenon where a patient fails to perceive something clearly present. Hallucinations, where something is perceived that is not there, are far more familiar and form a cornerstone of psychosis diagnosis.

When a patient shows they can neither hear nor see me, it becomes apparent that something entirely different is happening. In the first part of this trilogy, co-written with Verplancke, I described a patient with Cotard's syndrome who claimed to have no brain or heart and insisted they were dead (de Kroon & Verplancke, 2017). This involved a misjudgment of their own existence or a vital part of their body—a partial negation of the self.

Most hallucinations concern the perception of objects or people outside oneself. When observable objects or individuals are not perceived, we speak of a negative hallucination.

The question arises: how is this possible, and how can we situate it within a theoretical framework? Answering this requires examining the long trajectory of human thought, which began not in psychiatry or medicine but in philosophy. From the pre-Socratics to modern thinkers like Zeno of Elea, Edmund Husserl, Maurice Merleau-Ponty, Henri Bergson, Michel Foucault, Jacques Lacan, and Freud, the notion of nothingness has played an essential role in Western thought. Though this list includes no women or psychologists, the focus here is on the place of nothingness in philosophy and how psychiatry addresses it.

Negative Hallucination in Western Thought

The idea of nothingness has occupied a significant place in Western thought, influencing the way psychiatry grapples with complex phenomena like negative hallucination. Systematic philosophical thinking in the West began with the pre-Socratics, who grappled with paradoxes and the limitations of human perception. For example, Zeno of Elea's paradox of the flying arrow demonstrates how thought can contradict perception. The arrow, in flight, occupies different definable positions in space at successive moments. At any given instant, it appears to be at rest. If it is always at rest in every moment, the paradox suggests that it does not move at all. Modern mathematics has resolved this paradox, but Zeno's thought experiment illustrates how thinking can negate time and motion, contradicting lived experience.

This contradiction is central to understanding negative hallucination, where perception operates under a different logic than the one governing reality.

In modern philosophy, nothingness has re-emerged as a central theme, evident in Schopenhauer's negative ontology, Heidegger's **nichtiges Nichts**, and Sartre's **L'Être et le Néant**. The Hamletian question, "to be or not to be," reflects humanity's perennial confrontation with death, where consciousness ends and nothingness reigns. Death signifies the ultimate void, a place where thought ceases. In contemporary times, belief in an eternal soul persists more as metaphor than literal truth.

Human contact with reality occurs through two primary paths: perception and symbolization, the latter often mediated by language or abstract constructs like mathematical formulas. Direct perception is immediate and unmediated, a state without reflective distance, as seen in catatonia, where the subject is "frozen" by the immediacy of their reality. However, human existence also relies on the capacity for symbolization, where language and abstraction allow us to mediate, reflect upon, and communicate our experiences.

The Role of Symbolization in Perception

Negative hallucination is intimately connected to the process of symbolization. The separation of the subject from its immediate experience creates a void that demands to be filled. This void gives rise to language, introduced by the Other, who provides the material for the child's first acts of symbolization. Parents, for example, help the child fill this void with words, enabling the development of language and meaning-making.

However, the symbols offered by language are inherently "mere" representations, lacking the materiality of the things they signify. This gap between word and thing confirms the emptiness it attempts to fill. Conversely, if the child's emptiness is addressed solely with material objects, such as food or toys, without the introduction of language, the child may fail to develop symbolic capacities. The void, or absence, is a necessary condition for the emergence of language and the ability to symbolize.

Phenomenology and the Negative Hallucination

What does phenomenology have to say about negative hallucination? Maurice Merleau-Ponty, the philosopher of perception, does not directly address negative hallucination in his Phenomenology of Perception. However, he discusses positive hallucination, which involves perceiving phenomena or objects that do not exist in objective reality.

Merleau-Ponty analyses clinical reports of hallucinating patients and concludes: "Since the hallucination is not a sensory content, there is nothing left but to consider it as a judgement, as an interpretation or as a belief" (Merleau-Ponty, p. 434). Despite this, he argues that an intellectualized theory of hallucination is impossible, asking: "On what basis do empiricism and intellectualism fail to understand hallucination, and by what other method can we arrive at such an understanding?"

Merleau-Ponty critiques empiricism for attempting to explain hallucination as an over-stimulation of nerve centers, a view that presupposes the primacy of objective thought and reduces the hallucination to a physiological malfunction. He notes: "In this way, they falsify its own nature and its immanent sense; according to the sick themselves, the hallucination does not have its place in the objective being" (p. 435).

Intellectualism, on the other hand, assumes that hallucination arises from thought or consciousness, suggesting that the mind constructs and possesses its own experiences. This view fails to account for the psychotic inability to distinguish between reality and illusion, highlighting the limitations of both doctrines.

Returning to the Clinic

Reflecting on Melanie's case, it becomes clear that her negative hallucination illustrates gaps in perception and consciousness. She denied the existence of parts of her reality, a phenomenon that might be understood as a manifestation of the unconscious. Her experience demonstrates that perception is not a mere registration of objective reality but a human faculty centered on the subject.

The clinic, with its extreme cases of psychopathology, offers unique insights into the complexities of human perception. Melanie's case challenges the mechanistic approach prevalent in contemporary psychiatry, which treats symptoms as mechanical malfunctions to be eliminated. This reductionist view fails to address the subjective dimension of human experience. Psychopathology reminds us that the subjective cannot be discarded as unscientific; doing so compromises the very essence of good medicine.

The Role of Absence

The black hole of nothingness is everywhere: in the clinic, in science, and within the subject. Despite modern science's claim to unify mind and body, the chasm between the two persists. Science often overlooks or denies this void, leading to the question: is this oversight a negative hallucination or deliberate blindness?

Taking Lacan's adage, "Écoutez bien le malade" ("Listen closely to the patient"), to heart, we can better understand these phenomena. Melanie's case exemplifies how a gap in perception—a black hole in consciousness—can be associated with negative hallucination.

Moving Forward

As with previous chapters on Capgras and Cotard's syndromes, Melanie's case presents a phenomenon of absence. Capgras syndrome involves the absence of identity; Cotard's syndrome denies the existence of vital organs or life itself. Melanie's case, however, concerns the denial of something present in reality.

Her imaginary merging with her mirror image complicates her ability to separate and differentiate. This imaginary constellation creates difficulties in her relationships, work, and family life. Yet within the hospital ward, where staff place less demand on her subjectivity, she finds respite. In art therapy, she begins to depict her life story in labyrinthine drawings, reflecting her struggle to escape her impasse. Upon admission, she felt metaphorically dead, but now it seems she is on a path to resolution.

The child's initial identification with the libidinal subject is rooted in the imaginary order, comprising images and emotions. Early experiences are fragmented, and the child cannot distinguish between self and other, inside and outside. The body is experienced as a collection of separate parts (corps morcelé). Without symbolic correction, this fragmented identity may persist, leading to the projection of uncertainty onto others or the self. Entering the symbolic order through language involves the trauma of losing part of the self.

The Role of Symbolic Correction

The transition from the imaginary order to the symbolic order, where language and representation take precedence, is essential for the development of a cohesive sense of self. Without this symbolic correction, the fragmented experience of identity in the imaginary order may lead to pathological manifestations, such as the doppelganger phenomenon or the doubling of one's own self.

In Melanie's case, the absence of symbolic correction seems to have resulted in her inability to distinguish fully between herself and others, as well as a failure to reconcile her fragmented self-image. This lack of integration manifests in her behaviors, relationships, and the experience of negative hallucinations.

The process of entering the symbolic order is inherently traumatic, as it involves the loss of direct immediacy with oneself and the world. The symbolic introduces structure and meaning, but it also creates a void where unity once existed. This void may remain unresolved in some cases, perpetuating a fragmented sense of self and difficulties in integrating one's identity with reality.

Hallucination and Its Implications

To place the negative hallucination within the broader context of perception, it is important to revisit its phenomenological and psychoanalytic underpinnings. Negative hallucinations involve not just a gap in perception but a gap in meaning. This is different from ordinary misperceptions, as the missing element cannot be recovered through correction or reasoning.

For Melanie, the negative hallucination exemplifies her broader struggle with identity, symbolization, and integration into the symbolic order. Her inability to perceive aspects of reality reflects an absence in her psychic structure—a void that has yet to be filled through language and relational understanding.

In this sense, the negative hallucination can be understood as a breakdown in the process of symbolization. While the symbolic order allows us to name, define, and organize our experiences, its absence leaves the subject stranded in the imaginary realm, where fragmented and unstructured perceptions dominate. This inability to organize experiences into coherent narratives is evident in Melanie's art therapy, where her labyrinthine drawings reflect her struggle to navigate her fragmented internal world.

Implications for Psychiatry

Melanie's case highlights the limitations of the current mechanistic paradigm in psychiatry. This model prioritizes the elimination of symptoms through pharmacological and behavioral interventions, often at the expense of exploring the subjective and phenomenological aspects of the patient's experience.

The DSM-5, with its emphasis on categorization and symptom reduction, offers little insight into the deeper structures of psychopathology, particularly phenomena like negative hallucination. The overwhelming administrative burden in contemporary psychiatry further detracts from clinicians' ability to engage meaningfully with their patients.

To truly understand and address complex cases like Melanie's, psychiatry must reclaim its roots in phenomenology and psychoanalysis. These disciplines emphasize the subjective dimension of human experience, recognizing that the psyche cannot simply be reduced to the organic.

Nothingness and Its Philosophical Roots

The phenomenon of nothingness has deep roots in Western thought, beginning with the Book of Genesis, which posits that God created the heavens and the earth from a state of nothingness. This narrative underscores the foundational role of absence in human understanding of creation and existence.

Nothingness is not merely an abstract concept but a concrete aspect of human experience, as seen in the existential void encountered in moments of profound emptiness or loss. Philosophers like Heidegger and Sartre have explored this theme extensively, connecting nothingness to the human condition, consciousness, and the inevitability of death.

In Melanie's case, her experience of nothingness manifests through the negative hallucination—a perceptual and existential void that reflects the gaps in her psychic structure. This absence is not merely a sensory phenomenon but a symbolic one, tied to her struggles with identity, separation, and integration into the symbolic order.

Conclusion

Melanie's case provides a window into the complex interplay between perception, symbolization, and the subjective experience of reality. Her negative hallucination illustrates the profound impact of gaps in perception and meaning on the psyche, challenging the reductionist approaches of modern psychiatry.

By reconnecting with phenomenology and psychoanalysis, psychiatry can move beyond its current mechanistic paradigm to better understand and address the subjective dimensions of human experience. Melanie's case serves as a reminder that the subjective cannot be ignored without compromising the essence of psychiatric care.

As Lacan reminds us: "Écoutez bien le malade"—listen closely to the patient. Their stories, struggles, and gaps in perception hold the key to understanding the deeper structures of the human mind. In Melanie's labyrinthine drawings, we see not just a representation of her fragmented world but also the potential for healing and integration through the therapeutic process.

Further Thoughts on Nothingness in Psychosis

The transition into the Symbolic order marks a crucial developmental step. It is through language that the subject gains access to meaning, structure, and differentiation. However, this transition comes at a cost: the loss of an immediate, Imaginary unity and the confrontation with a symbolic framework that imposes rules, limitations, and separations. The trauma of this entry lies in the realization that the subject is no longer whole but split—divided between the Real, the Imaginary, and the Symbolic.

The Symbolic order enables the subject to establish an identity, but this identity is mediated through the Other, who provides the names, categories, and roles that structure the subject's world. This "alienating identification" ensures that the subject's sense of self is both given by and dependent on the Other. The price for this structuring is alienation: the subject's self-perception is no longer purely internal but mediated by external representations.

For patients like ours, the failure to fully enter the Symbolic order results in a fragile or fragmented sense of self. Without a clear distinction between self and Other, the patient remains trapped in the Imaginary, where merging, duplication, and identification dominate. The mirror image becomes more than a reflection; it becomes a presence, a *phantasm* that erases the boundaries of individuality. This inability to separate oneself from the reflection reflects a failure to achieve *symbolic castration*—the necessary loss that opens the subject to the symbolic dimension of meaning and structure.

In the clinic, we see how these dynamics play out. The patient's drawings, labyrinthine and sprawling, symbolize her internal experience: a maze with no clear exit, a struggle to achieve coherence and separation. Her question—"How do I get out of this impasse?"—captures the existential dilemma of a subject unable to navigate the transition from the Imaginary to the Symbolic. The hospital environment, by minimizing direct appeals to her subjectivity, provides temporary relief, but it does not resolve the underlying problem.

Art therapy serves as a bridge, allowing the patient to express her experience in a form that precedes language yet gestures toward it. The drawings act as intermediaries, visual representations of her fragmented self and her attempts to reconstitute it. They offer a space where the Imaginary can be externalized, observed, and, eventually, symbolized.

In cases like this, clinical practice must carefully mediate the transition into the Symbolic order. Too forceful an appeal to the patient's subjectivity risks exacerbating her confusion and resistance. Instead, the therapeutic process must proceed gradually, providing a space for the Imaginary to unfold while gently introducing elements of the Symbolic. By working through the images and narratives that dominate her experience, the patient can begin to establish a coherent sense of self and navigate the trauma of symbolic entry.

PART 4

Towards a Different Perspective of the Subject

Introduction

Science often seeks to remove subjectivity, aiming for pure objectivity, but in psychiatry this is neither possible nor desirable. Without the subject, psychiatry loses its meaning. Even in science, subjectivity creeps in, as Heisenberg's uncertainty principle shows. Psychiatry, if it is to be a true human science, must make space for the subjective dimension. Structuralism offers a way to integrate the subject into human science without reducing mind to body. Mind and body influence one another, yet they belong to different orders and need not be forced into a false unity. Looking from a parallax perspective allows both to coexist without demanding resolution.

The French writer Georges Perec once composed a novel without the letter "e", a constraint that both conceals and reveals an absence. This echoes Lacan's concept of the objet petit a, an imagined remnant of what is missing, originating in the separation from the Other at psychic birth. Desire is rooted in this lack, just as Freud's theories were animated by a longing to connect psyche and soma. Lacan, unlike Freud, was not bound to biological explanations; he explored the interplay of the Real, the Imaginary, and the Symbolic, with desire sustained by sublimation through language.

The idea of nothingness plays a central role in both philosophy and psychiatry. Sartre questioned whether being or non-being comes first, seeing being as primary but unable to define non-being clearly. In psychological development, separations—first imaginary, then symbolic—create the foundations for identity. In the mirror stage, the child begins to imagine

DOI: 10.4324/9781003675389-14

the Other's presence even in absence, which fosters the ability to symbolise. Without complete separation, hallucinations and delusions can emerge, functioning as defences against the abyss of non-being. Some patients live close to this void, as in nihilistic delusions, where the protective shield of language collapses entirely. The variations of human desire are endless, from exploration and art to intimate relationships, yet encounters with nothingness—whether in mental illness or in events like suicide—remind us of its unsettling proximity.

The mind–body problem remains unresolved. Neuroscience has encouraged a monistic view, equating mental life with brain function, yet this cannot explain consciousness or free thought. If such phenomena were purely neuronal, machines would possess them, but they do not. Consciousness is tied to the body in life, but this does not prove the existence of an immortal soul. The history of the word "psyche", rooted in Greek notions of breath, life force, and spirit, shows that it has always meant more than the brain's workings. The evolutionary and developmental emergence of self-awareness reflects a complex interplay of biology, language, and cultural structures.

Reductionist approaches, especially in Anglo-Saxon traditions, tend to collapse the mind into the brain, but philosophers such as Searle and Chalmers have challenged this, insisting that subjective experience resists such simplification. Chalmers' suggestion that information might equal consciousness risks conflating symbolic meaning with material carriers, a category error. Classical psychiatry distinguished between levels of consciousness and its content, recognising that the qualitative aspects belong more to psychiatry and psychology than to neurology. The challenge remains: no physical substrate has been found for qualitative consciousness. For now, the problem seems beyond our current modes of thought.

Lacan's model highlights two prerequisites for subjectivity: immersion in the symbolic order of language, and separation from the primary other, usually the mother. The "Name-of-the-Father" disrupts the original symbiosis, enabling the child to enter language and culture, where desire is endlessly renewed because words can never fully coincide with the Real. If these processes fail, the individual's relationship with reality and their own body can become profoundly distorted, as in psychotic syndromes where symbolic meaning collapses and reality is reinterpreted in ways that defy consensus.

The absence of a physical marker for psychosis undermines the purely biological paradigm that dominates modern psychiatry. Neuroleptics can calm and stabilise, but they do not address the essence of psychosis. The core delusions often remain untouched, even if hallucinations are somewhat reduced. Their side effects—ranging from movement disorders to severe fatigue—can be distressing enough for patients to stop taking them. Medication can be useful, but it should be prescribed cautiously, in dialogue with the patient, and not in a rigid attempt to eradicate all symptoms. High doses often diminish quality of life without truly resolving psychosis.

Psychosis is mainly anarrative phenomenon. People experiencing it often have stories to tell, yet these are frequently dismissed or ignored. Without contact and recognition, isolation deepens. Many professionals retreat into administrative tasks or protective distance, leaving patients lonelier still. Some nurses, however, approach patients with an intuitive humanity that bypasses clinical detachment, engaging with them as people rather than cases. Simple acts of inclusion—offering meaningful activities, involving patients in community efforts—can restore a sense of belonging, as seen when withdrawn patients suddenly rallied to help during a flood.

Understanding psychosis requires moving beyond the assumption that only somatic treatments matter. Psychiatry must resist becoming an entirely mechanistic practice. Structuralism offers an alternative vision: one that recognises the gap between word and thing, denotation and connotation, and sees this gap not as a flaw but as the source of creativity, connection, and freedom of thought. Modern psychiatry's obsession with denotative thinking—reducing patients to diagnostic categories—risks suffocating the very subject it seeks to understand.

This alternative approach does not romanticise psychosis, but it refuses to strip it of meaning. Psychotic experiences may seem alien and illogical, yet they arise within symbolic and personal contexts that can be explored through dialogue. To work effectively with psychosis, practitioners must leave the safety of rigid protocols, tolerate uncertainty, and meet patients where they are. This involves listening deeply, not to decode pathology but to build a bridge between the patient's subjective world and the shared symbolic order. Language plays a central role in this process, as in psychosis the structures that normally organise reality may fragment, making shared meaning difficult but not impossible. Both the other and the Other play a vital role in the therapeutic relationship.

Structuralism also restores the social and cultural context to psychiatry. Psychotic experiences are shaped not only by individual history but by the broader symbolic networks in which people live. This challenges the dominance of biological reductionism, reminding us that brain chemistry is only one thread in the complex fabric of mental life. Therapy, then, becomes not simply about symptom control but about re-establishing connections—to others, to language, to the self.

In practice, this means creating spaces where people with psychosis can speak freely, without fear of dismissal. It means resisting the temptation to treat the mind as a machine and patients as faulty components. It means valuing the richness of subjective experience and the creative possibilities of dialogue. Such an approach requires both intellectual openness and emotional resilience. It asks the therapist to acknowledge their own strangeness, their own encounters with emptiness, so that they can meet the patient without the shield of clinical distance.

Psychiatry's future depends on its capacity to evolve beyond its current fixation on objectivity and control. The move from denotative to connotative thinking is not just a theoretical exercise; it is a moral imperative. To reduce patients to symptoms is to deny their humanity. A structuralist approach restores that humanity, placing the subject at the heart of the therapeutic encounter. It asks us to see psychosis not only as an illness but as a particular way of being in the world, one that demands understanding as much as treatment. This is not easy work, but it is the work that matters most.

By embracing the interplay between language, desire, and meaning, psychiatry can become not merely a branch of medicine but a truly human science. It can shed its denotative straitjacket and recover its capacity for curiosity, compassion, and genuine engagement. In doing so, it may finally move closer to understanding the psyche—not as a puzzle to be solved, but as a living, speaking subject whose depth cannot be exhausted by any one theory or method.

10

SUBJECT AND SCIENCE

Science's inherent focus on objectivity often excludes subjectivity as much as possible, fostering a discourse that risks becoming hermetically sealed. Psychiatry, on the other hand, targets the whole person, necessitating an engagement with the subject. This creates significant challenges for psychiatry as it seeks credibility as a scientific discipline while addressing the inherent tension between subject and object. A dialectical stance, as suggested in Chapter 5 (Nothingness and Science), offers a potential resolution, embracing opposition without succumbing to reductive synthesis. In this sense, the dialectic between word and thing and between the symbolic and the real has no final stage.

Science aspires to be objective and excludes subjectivity as much as possible. In psychiatry, however, this is impossible. By excluding the subject, psychiatry becomes a dead letter. Even in science, subjectivity creeps in, as demonstrated by Heisenberg's uncertainty principle. Why should psychiatry be any different? If psychiatry is to be a true human science, it must make room for the subject. Through structuralism, the integration of the subject into (human) science becomes possible.

It may be too much to claim that structuralism can resolve the mind–body problem, but reducing the psyche to the soma is simply untrue. It is probably best to allow both to coexist with their own distinct identities. Certainly, soma and psyche influence one another, but they belong to different orders. Both can be considered from a *parallax view*, as Žižek, 2006 calls it, thereby postponing the need for an integration or resolution (*epoche*).

In 1969, the experimental writer Georges Perec published a curious novel that lacks the letter "e," the most common letter in the French

DOI: 10.4324/9781003675389-15

language. The title of this e-less novel is *La Disparition* (The Disappearance). The Dutch translation follows the same constraint, also omitting the letter "e" from the text. In Dutch, "e" is likewise the most common vowel. The translation of the title as *The Manco* effectively captures the essence of the novel: something is missing. The story is both captivating and profound. The main character, Anton Vocalis, experiences a unique sense of absence that he seeks to understand but cannot fully grasp. Others join in this search for what is missing, and during their investigations, it becomes evident that the family is cursed. As soon as a character realizes what is happening, they die, as naming the absence of the letter "e" is a transgression punishable by death. The characters in the novel are condemned to live with the absence of the letter "e." Perec's underlying motivation for this story is the loss of his mother, who was murdered in Auschwitz.

This scenario in Perec's work strongly resembles Lacan's concept of the *objet petit a*. The *objet petit a* is primarily an imaginary representation of something that is missing. It refers to the Other, from whom the subject is separated at psychic birth. It signifies something that is no longer there, an absence that simultaneously exerts a powerful attraction. Desire is rooted in this lack—the driving force behind all human life. It is the immaterial equivalent of Freud's concept of instinct. Freud was deeply entrenched in the biological paradigm of his time, aspiring to establish a scientific foundation for psychoanalysis. In his "fictions," he frequently expressed a desire to explain psychological mechanisms in somatic terms, though he was never able to fulfill this aspiration. For Freud, it remained an unfulfilled longing. This limitation proved to be a strength, as it allowed him to create fictions and constructs that became the foundation of the psychoanalytic framework. His internal conflict gave rise to a body of thought that has benefited many.

Lacan, unlike Freud, was not bound by a preference for biological explanatory models. Instead, he pursued a more transcendent approach while maintaining a connection to the Real. Some aspects of his thought remain obscure, and the *objet petit a* is one such example. While the *objet petit a* refers to the Other, of which it is a part, it also disappears, leaving nothing behind. Our imagination fills this void with remnants such as feces, the gaze, and the voice. When the *objet petit a* takes on tangible qualities, desire is reduced to needs, which can be satisfied, thus approaching death—the cessation of desire, equated with death itself. Desire must persist as long as one avoids the inherent danger of the Real. To navigate this danger, humans have invented sublimation, which, at its best, can be achieved through symbolization, realized in language.

As noted earlier, parallels can be drawn between philosophy and psychiatric practice concerning the concept of the negative. Philosophers often address the ontology of being and non-being, while psychiatry focuses on exploring the psychological underpinnings of the negative in psychopathology. Sartre, for instance, ponders whether being or non-being comes first. According to Sartre, being is primary and does not precede nothingness. Non-being is not derivative of being (Sartre, 1943). However, Sartre struggles to define what non-being actually is.

In my view, non-being is an effect of processes within being, subject to the constraints of time. Understanding this requires consideration of human psychological development. At psychic birth, the subject undergoes two separations: the first imaginary and the second symbolic. Lacan elaborates on these separations—described as "castrations"—in his theories of the "mirror stage" and the "Law-of-the-Father" (Lacan, 1946, 1949). During the mirror stage, triggered by real circumstances, the young child begins to separate from the mother. When the mother leaves the room, the child experiences anxiety and cries. Upon the mother's return, the child reacts with joy. The child sees its reflection in the face of the Other and eventually learns to imagine the Other's presence even in their absence, giving rise to positive hallucination.

These processes of separation, as well as imaginary and symbolic identification, grant immense freedom in the realms of imagination and meaning-making. In this stage, there is no distinction between fiction and reality. The absence of boundaries allows the psychotic to indulge in limitless imaginings, unchecked by any law. Only common sense could potentially restrain them.

When the process of separation is incomplete, the child may persist in imagining the object of their desire (the mother), which could manifest as a hallucination. Similarly, disruptions in the symbolization process can lead to delusions. A psychotic individual, experiencing the absence of being, exists outside the dialectic of being and non-being, positioned instead on the side of failure. Whether this state is compatible with life is questionable. Typically, delusions or hallucinations act as defense mechanisms, preventing the individual from fully succumbing to the void of non-being—what is referred to as *horror vacui*.

The aforementioned considerations resonate with Wouter Kusters' ideas in his *Philosophy of Madness*. As an experienced expert in this field, Kusters offers insights that bring him closer to the source of these experiences than I can claim to be (Kusters, 2020).

If we now relate these considerations about nothingness—as explored through the three experiences of nothingness outlined in Chapters 7–9—to nihilistic delusions and negative hallucinations, we must conclude that the filling of this "nothing" is artificial and highly variable. The ways in which human desire manifests itself are inexhaustible, like the shifting patterns of a kaleidoscope. We imagine and pursue journeys to the moon and Mars, create breathtaking works of art, and write extraordinary stories. Yet sometimes, we are startled when someone confronts the abyss of nothingness—such as when a loved one commits suicide. Similarly, patients may recount their experiences of confronting nothingness, offering insights into realities most of us instinctively avoid. The question remains whether these patients, particularly those with nihilistic delusions or negative hallucinations, are still shielded from the full impact of this confrontation or whether they are already immersed within it.

In the clinical trilogy of nothingness, the *doppelgänger delusion* represents the mildest form of confrontation with nothingness. The negative hallucination brings the patient closer to the abyss, while the nihilistic delusion seems to fully engulf the individual. In the latter case, the protective shield of language that normally mediates between the subject and the Real has been entirely stripped away.

After 45 years of working with psychotic patients, I must admit that no medication—not even the best available treatments—has effectively "washed away" psychotic disorders. While agitation and anxiety can be alleviated, the core delusion remains unshaken. Maintaining contact with these patients is critical, as no person can endure the absolute isolation that psychosis entails. Some mental health professionals understand this and intentionally stay close to these individuals, providing essential support. Moreover, it is important to listen to psychotic patients because they often articulate truths that challenge or expand our understanding of the human condition.

The Mind–Body Debate: Challenges and Implications

The debate surrounding the mind–body problem continues to inspire philosophical, scientific, and clinical inquiry. With the rise of neuroscience, it might seem that the dualistic divide has been resolved, favoring a monistic view where the body reigns supreme. According to this perspective, psychological phenomena are entirely attributed to the brain and its neuronal processes, which are responsible for memory, thinking, and consciousness. However, even the staunchest proponents of this physicalist view cannot fully explain certain fundamental aspects of the human mind, such as the existence of consciousness and the freedom of thought.

If consciousness and thought were solely functions of neural networks, then artificial systems such as robots or computers would presumably possess these qualities. Yet they do not. While machines can simulate cognitive processes, they lack the relational, subjective, and symbolic dimensions that define human consciousness. The cessation of life—marked by the absence of *res cogitans*—reveals that consciousness is intricately tied to the body. However, this observation does not necessarily imply the existence of an immortal soul.

Etymological and Mythological Origins of "Psyche"

To gain a deeper understanding of the concept of the psyche, an etymological and mythological exploration is illuminating. The word "psyche" derives from the Greek *psuchè* (ψυχή), which refers not only to the soul but also to breath, life force, and spirit. The mythological figure Psyche, described in Apuleius' *Metamorphoses*, is a beautiful princess who, after a series of trials and adventures, marries the god Eros (Apuleius, n.d. Together, they have a daughter named Hedone (Pleasure in Greek, Voluptas in Latin) (Rey, 1995).

The Greek verb *psuchein* (ψύχειν) means "to give life" or "to enliven." Similarly, the noun "psychosis" denotes a process of animating or giving life (Van Veen, 1991). Originally, *psyche* comes from the verb *psycho* (ψύχω), meaning "to blow" or "to cool by blowing." The term encompasses various aspects of vitality and spirit, including courage, intellect, and willpower (Müller & Thiel, 1958). In essence, the word "psyche" connects to all vital functions and, metonymically, points to the individual as a subject.

This rich history underscores the inadequacy of equating the psyche solely with the brain or its neural functions. While thoughts and consciousness undoubtedly involve the brain, reducing them entirely to neurophysiological processes oversimplifies the complexity of human experience.

Evolution, Self-Awareness, and the Emergence of Consciousness

Tracing the historical and evolutionary roots of the mind–body problem reveals intriguing possibilities. Modern thinkers like Michel Foucault have argued that significant shifts in the status of the subject have occurred throughout history (Foucault, 1966). These cultural and philosophical transformations pale in comparison to the profound evolutionary leaps that gave rise to human self-awareness over millions of years.

Ontogeny, the development of the individual, reflects phylogeny, the evolution of the species. Observing the psychological development of a child offers a microcosmic view of humanity's broader journey toward self-awareness. Each step in a child's development—from the mirror stage to language acquisition—represents a revolutionary transformation. Yet these same transformative processes are fraught with potential disruptions, underscoring the delicate balance required for the emergence of a cohesive sense of self.

Could the acquisition of a psyche be explained merely as an evolutionary survival mechanism? Perhaps. Yet the human capacity for self-awareness, imagination, and desire also carries the potential for destructive behaviors, such as genocide and war. These phenomena challenge the simplistic notion that the psyche exists solely as a tool for survival.

Critiques of Reductionism: A Broader Perspective

In the Anglo-Saxon tradition, the mind–body problem has often been approached with skepticism or outright dismissal. Many philosophers reduce the issue to a one-dimensional framework, equating mind with the physical functions of the brain. However, this reductionism has met significant criticism from figures such as John Searle and David Chalmers.

Searle asserts that consciousness cannot be reduced to physical processes alone (Searle, 1992). Chalmers, while open to the possibility of dualism, critiques reductive models for failing to account for subjective experience (Chalmers, 1996). He emphasizes "experience" as the cornerstone of his argument, connecting it to consciousness, language, and information processing. Chalmers convincingly demonstrates that reductionism cannot resolve the relationship between body and mind, as experience and consciousness are properties of the subject that transcend neuro-physical explanations.

In his most recent work, *Reality+*, Chalmers proposes that information equals consciousness and claims that a "bit" of information is a physical thing (Chalmers, 2022). However, this hypothesis reduces the symbolic to the material, a reduction that constitutes a formal error in scientific reasoning. A bit, at most, is a carrier of information with both material and symbolic dimensions. These dimensions belong to fundamentally different orders and cannot be conflated.

In classical psychiatry, the researcher employed a research theme in clinical practice, wherein consciousness was assessed in addition to mood and conative functions.[1] A distinction was made between a quantitative aspect and a qualitative aspect. The quantitative part corresponds to what neurologists also reference in their research of the central nervous system. The levels of consciousness distinguished are as follows: compos mentis (clear consciousness), reduced attention, somnolence (drowsiness), sopor (continuous sinking), stupor (gaining consciousness briefly with numerous painful stimuli), and coma (being completely unconscious). Sometimes syncope (a short period of coma) is included in this classification.[2] These stages describe clarity and are separate from the content of consciousness. The content of consciousness is of an entirely different order and, in fact, encompasses the whole range of thoughts and images. When the thought contents are considered in the light of psychopathological classification, one may use most of the DSM-5, which I do not recommend to anyone; it is better to utilize the classic psychiatric classification. In this framework, there can be neurosis, psychosis, and perversions, the latter corresponding to personality disorders.

What Solms is aiming for is precisely the neurological aspect of consciousness, which he situates in the brainstem where vital functions are mediated. The qualitative part lies just outside of that and is actually the domain of psychiatry and psychology, or at least it should be.

There are those, like Eric Kandel, who believe that psychiatry and neurology should reunite. To justify this view, he first proposed the idea that the psyche is a biological function (Kandel, 2018). This far-reaching reductionism has since become common in psychiatry, and in psychoanalysis there are also proponents of this idea. I think this perspective is more about belief than science. I suspect that phenomenologists are somewhat more cautious in this matter, appealing to their assumption of the epochè, the suspension of judgment on the issue.

The major problem in this field is that no substrate has been identified for qualitative consciousness. This fact has been highlighted by Chalmers, Nagel, and Searle, thinkers who belong to the Anglo-Saxon tradition. The continental tradition of thought on this problem generally adopts a much more reserved and nuanced stance than is the case in Anglo-Saxon circles.

The question remains whether a solution to this fundamental problem can be found in the future. It does not seem possible with our current modes of thinking. There are those who argue that perhaps a higher level of intelligence is required to tackle the mind–body problem. The solutions currently proposed resemble the proverbial bull in a china shop, where the problem is simply dismissed by asserting either that there is no problem at all and that it is an illusion or that the psyche is reduced to the body, which perhaps amounts to the same thing. To use a metaphor: they equate a Mozart symphony with the holes in a CD disc.

Researchers working with artificial intelligence (AI) are also generally more cautious about taking a strong position in this mind–body debate. So far, I have observed that they believe robots do not possess self-awareness.

The researchers working on quantum computers are primarily focused on achieving even greater capacities for these machines, but there is something fundamentally different about quantum computers that distinguishes them from conventional devices. The binary principle has been surpassed in quantum computers. A signal is no longer simply on or off; it can be both on and off simultaneously. This development will have significant consequences for computer science, but I doubt whether it will solve the mind–body problem.

Desire and Symbolization

In Lacanian terms, the patient with negative hallucinations described in Chapter 9 has not moved beyond imaginary existence as the sole mode of experience, a situation in which she still coincides with her mirror image, a world of inseparability. She has evaded the trauma of the cleavage, as a result of which desire has not been able to take root. Desire, which can only express itself through language, appears to fail whenever words are used, as they struggle to overcome inseparability or at least attempt to do so. The longing for that inseparability remains and is nourished by the imaginary identification with one's own reflection. The symbolic shield of language conceals the trauma of separation, but at the same time, the traumatic event actualizes the impossibility of inseparability.

It is evident that the other plays a crucial role in this dynamic. If this other person is not themselves split/separated, then they will regard the child as an imaginary filler for their own deficiency. The child seduces the other into this symbiotic constellation where no words are spoken, and mother and child (the mother usually being the first other) feast upon one another to avoid the trauma of separation.

When the subject, upon entering the symbolic world, is separated from a part of itself, a memory persists of the idea that lack or separation has been eradicated. The longing for that paradisiacal state always endures. In the split subject, the phantasm of an unseparated being persists in desire. The separation, also referred to as castration, occurs through the intervention of a third term, represented by the father. In the Oedipal constellation, he disrupts the symbiotic relationship between mother and child, enabling the child-subject to begin an autonomous life and redirecting the mother's love toward her partner.

Considerations

In Chapters 3 and 4, we described the structuring role of language and, in Chapter 5, the psychological development of the child during the mirror stage and the symbolic stage. Here, we revisit the normal development of the child in light of the structuring of the subject, whereby a certain identity is established. A strong reliance is placed on Lacan's teachings. At least two factors are crucial here: an environment in which people speak and where laws govern human interactions. This structure is commonly referred to as the "Other." The second factor concerns separation. This occurs not only in the physical reality between mother and child but also on a more fundamental level between word and thing. Word and thing are distinct entities that cannot be reduced to one another. There is a tension between word and thing that is insoluble and is reactivated each time a word is spoken.

The two components required to undergo the symbolization process discussed above are examined here in more detail. First, the symbolization process involves an environment in which the symbolic exerts its influence—namely, the world of language. The symbolic can essentially be traced back to language with its grammatical and syntactic structure, as well as its metaphorical and metonymic functions. Language also has a specific structure and operates according to its own logic and laws.

Meaning emerges from the complex interplay of signs in their mutual relationships. At least two signifiers are required to generate meaning. In psychoanalytic discourse, the signifier (e.g., a word) has the characteristic of condensation, as with metaphor and symptom. The signified represents the shift, the metonymy (Saussure, 1916; de Kroon, 1993). Metaphor and metonymy are figures of speech that generate meaning in their own unique ways. A metaphor is a figure of speech based on a simile that should not be taken literally. Examples include: "He has elephant skin" and "We were overwhelmed with data by a tsunami." A metonymy is a figure of speech in which an image shift occurs; instead of the intended, something associated with the intended is mentioned. An example is: "The fleet has seven sails." In this example, there is a dividing line between sail and boat. Both metaphor and metonymy possess a negativity, an inability to fully represent the intended object. This inability simultaneously constitutes the richness of language. Symptoms behave like metaphors and metonymies in their inability as well as in their richness and diversity. In psychiatric practice, interpreting these in their context is both a challenge and an art.

The linguistic structures and mechanisms outlined above adhere to laws underlying human communication, the creation of meaning in the world around us, and the understanding of one's own body. This latter aspect is particularly important for our identity as subjects. It is not without reason that Lacan asserted that the subject is an effect of language (Lacan, 1966).

The second component necessary to arrive at subjectivity is separation—separation from the primary other, usually the mother, as outlined in Chapter 5. This developmental process is described here using the Oedipus constellation. This is the Oedipal triangle involving the child, the mother, and the father figure. Initially, there is a symbiotic relationship between mother and child, characterized by inertia. There is no impetus for the child to move beyond this, and the same tendency exists in the mother. However, her situation is somewhat more complex. If her own development has been unproblematic, she has already entered the symbolic order and, moreover, has a partner to whom she should direct her love. The child cannot be everything to her, as this is incompatible with life for both herself and the child, particularly psychic life. A caesura must therefore be enacted in the symbiotic relationship. This task falls to the third element in the Oedipal triangle, the father. He must disrupt the close relationship between mother and child, ensuring the mother redirects her attention and love to him. This intrusive act frees the child from the mother's suffocating embrace. Lacan refers to this violent act as castration (Lacan, 1966). Through this separation, the child develops the desire to return to the initial state of nirvana in the womb, where no tension existed.

We are all familiar with desire, and according to Lacan, it is ideally expressed in language. Other forms of expression may give shape to desire but lack the sublime[3] capacity of language. This set of interactive processes within the Oedipal constellation and its laws is termed by Lacan as "Le Nom-du-Père," the "Name-of-the-Father" (Lacan, 1966). Some forms of satisfying desire have decidedly perverse[4] characteristics, especially when desire is mistaken for needs satisfied in various ways.

With the expression of desire in language, something occurs that sustains desire. Each word spoken proves insufficient to fulfil the desire. On the contrary, language actualizes desire because words do not coincide with what they express in the Real. Here too, there is a fundamental rift, which is constitutive for speech and culture. Speech propels itself forward, forming a chain of words that never ends unless one is dead.

These two components—the pre-existing language provided by the Other, with which the child identifies, and castration—are the prerequisites for becoming a speaking being and participating in the cultural environment. Through these processes, the speaking being is able to relate symbolically to the reality they inhabit and also to symbolize their own body. This process is accompanied by the emergence of consciousness, with its counterpart in the unconscious.

If something goes fundamentally wrong with the integration of the meaning system within the subject, it has severe consequences for their relationship with reality and their own body. This is evident in paranoia, where the relationship to other people and the world in general is disrupted, as well as in the relationship to one's own body. In the latter case, the assignment of meaning can lead to distorted interpretations, as described in this text regarding Cotard's syndrome (de Kroon & Verplancke, 2017, in this volume) and Capgras syndrome. The symbolic system becomes completely unbalanced, and the signifiers become attached to interpretations that bear no relation to reality. In Cotard's syndrome, this manifests as the belief that one has no heart, lungs, or brain, or is dead. In Capgras syndrome, it manifests as the belief that another person is not the real other but a doppelgänger.

Notes

1 The conative functions are understood to mean the faculties of the subject's will. Apathy is a lack of emotions, motivation, or enthusiasm. In aboulia, there is a lack of willpower. These disorders can occur with all kinds of psychiatric and somatic problems. In psychiatry it usually occurs in depression and psychoses, when negative symptomatology is particularly at play.
2 See also the Glasgow coma scale (https://www.wikiwand.com/en/Glasgow_Coma_Scale).
3 In Lacan's mind, this is a difficult passage. The sublime is directly related to sublimation. Sublimation functions as a socially accepted escape from an excess of sexual energy that can lead to socially unacceptable forms of discharge such as perverted behavior or neurotic symptoms. At least that's how Freud thought about it. Lacan connects sublimation with his ethics as described in his seventh Séminaire (Lacan, 1959–1960). First of all, Lacan does not regard the drives as natural phenomena in which energy is discharged, but as linguistic phenomena. Related to this, Lacan says that sublimation is never complete because the word never fully reaches the Thing. In sublimation, the subject does not change its object, but the object is given a different place in the symbolic system. Moreover, Lacan connects sublimation with the death instinct. The death drive is not only destructive but also a desire or will to create something out of nothing. And finally, the sublime object is the Thing that fascinates the subject. The Thing the psychotic is also looking for and becomes fascinated by his own imagination in the hallucination (cfr. Evans, 1996).
4 Perverse see the previous footnote. In this context, it is worth noting that Lacan perversely associates with the Law, the Name-of-the-Father. Perverse also means *vers le père*, against the father.

11

LOOKING FOR THE PSYCHE IN PSYCHIATRY

This chapter centers on Lacan's concept of the *objet petit a*, a residue of the separation process between mother and child. Though imperceptible, this "object" drives desire, symbolizing the yearning to restore lost unity. This dynamic aligns with structuralist insights regarding the separation between word and thing, as articulated in the Symbolic order. In psychosis, the distinct realms of the Real, Imaginary, and Symbolic become intertwined, manifesting in hallucinations and delusions.

The psyche is closely linked to the human ability to speak. This symbolic faculty is unique to humans. Plants and animals do not speak. Although they are capable of exchanging information through signals, this does not possess the symbolic capacity that characterizes human communication. This symbolic ability makes (self-)awareness possible.

Contrary to what is sometimes suggested today, Artificial Intelligence (AI) is not capable of generating consciousness.

For the above reasons, speech holds such a central place in psychiatry.

Lacan, in contrast, was not constrained by Freud's preference for biological explanatory models. He more closely followed the path of transcendence, without losing sight of the Real. Some aspects of Lacan's theories remain obscure, and the *objet petit a* is one such example. The *objet petit a* refers to the Other, of which it is a part, but it also disappears; nothing remains, and our imagination fills this void with reminiscences of feces, the gaze, and the voice. As soon as the *objet petit a* takes on tangible qualities, desire is replaced by needs, which can be satisfied. This, however, brings us closer to death, or the end of desire, which is equivalent to death. Desire must remain alive as long as we steer clear of the danger inherent in the Real.

DOI: 10.4324/9781003675389-16

To this end, humanity has invented sublimation, which, at its best, can be realized through symbolization, facilitated by language.

As we noted earlier, there are parallels between philosophy and psychiatric practice when it comes to exploring negativity. Philosophers often examine the ontology of being and non-being, while psychiatry focuses on the psychological roots of negativity in psychopathology. Sartre, for instance, asks which comes first: being or non-being. According to Sartre, being is primary and does not precede itself; non-being is not derived from being (Sartre, 1943). But what exactly is non-being? Sartre struggles to define it.

In my view, non-being is an effect of processes that unfold over time. Understanding this requires considering human psychological development. During psychic birth, the subject undergoes two separations: the first, imaginative; and the second, symbolic. Lacan elaborated on these separations (which he termed "castrations") in his theories of the "mirror stage" and the "Law-of-the-Father" (Lacan, 1946, 1949). In the mirror stage, the young child distances itself from the mother due to real circumstances. When the mother leaves the room, the child becomes anxious and cries. When she returns, the child beams with joy. Over time, the child learns to imagine the Other in her absence. This process gives birth to positive hallucination.

These separations and processes of imaginary and symbolic identification are accompanied by almost limitless freedom of imagination and meaning-making. Everything can be imagined and symbolized. The psychotic exploits this limitlessness, unrestrained by any laws or common sense that might otherwise keep them grounded. If the separation process falters, the child's imagined object of desire (the mother) may persist, resulting in hallucinations. Similarly, disruptions in the symbolization process can lead to delusions.

The psychotic who experiences the void of non-being is outside the dialectic of being and non-being; they exist on the side of failure. The question is whether this state is compatible with life. Hallucinations and delusions often serve as defense mechanisms against being completely engulfed by the black hole of non-being—what we might call *horror vacui*.

This line of thought aligns closely with Wouter Kusters' *Philosophy of Madness*. Kusters, as an expert by experience, is closer to the source than I am (Kusters, 2020).

When we relate these reflections on nothingness—particularly the three experiences of nothingness outlined in Chapters 7–9—with nihilistic delusion and negative hallucination, we conclude that the response to this void is always artificial, taking countless forms. Human desire manifests in endless variations: we fantasize about space travel, create breathtaking art, and write extraordinary stories. Yet we are sometimes shocked when someone confronts the abyss of nothingness directly, as in the case of suicide. Patients experiencing nihilistic delusions or negative hallucinations are not merely protected from this confrontation; they are often in the midst of it.

In the trilogy on clinical encounters with nothingness (Chapters 7–9), the doppelgänger delusion represents the mildest form of confrontation. Negative hallucination brings the patient closer to nothingness, while the nihilistic delusion seems to engulf them entirely. Here, the shield of language that protects against the Real is gone.

After 45 years of working with psychotics, I must admit that no medicine, not even the best, has been able to resolve psychotic disorders. Delusions persist despite mitigating unrest and fear. It is vital to maintain contact with these patients, as no one can endure the absolute isolation of psychosis. Some mental health professionals understand this and remain close to their patients. Listening to psychotic individuals is equally important, as they may tell us things we do not yet know.

The body–mind debate remains unresolved. While neuroscience seems to have won the battle for monism, problems remain—chiefly the existence of consciousness and freedom of thought. If these were merely products of neuronal networks, robots and computers would possess them too. This is clearly not the case. Consciousness and thought cannot simply be equated with the functions of the brain.

To equate thoughts and consciousness solely with brain functions is inadequate.

Modern human history, as Michel Foucault observes, has seen significant shifts in the status of the subject (Foucault, 1966). These changes are tiny compared to humanity's evolutionary strides toward self-awareness. This ontogenesis is mirrored in the child's development, which involves revolutionary steps toward self-awareness, shaped by interaction with the Other.

The reductionist view of consciousness as brain activity overlooks its phenomenological properties. Thinkers like David Chalmers acknowledge this complexity (Chalmers, 1996, 2022). His proposals, while promising, remain speculative. Future interdisciplinary collaboration may yet yield deeper insights.

Chalmers' argument, while speculative, invites engagement from other fields beyond neuroscience, such as linguistics, developmental psychology, and structuralism. However, the integration of these disciplines into a cohesive model remains a task for the future. In his latest book, *Reality+*, Chalmers posits that information equals consciousness (Chalmers, 2022). He further claims that a bit constitutes information and that a bit is a tangible thing. Taken together, these assertions imply that consciousness is inherently material.

This hypothesis, despite Chalmers' intellectual honesty, is one I cannot accept. The central issue lies in equating a bit with information. To me, a bit is merely an information carrier, comprising two aspects: the material and the symbolic. These two dimensions are fundamentally distinct. Reducing the symbolic to the material constitutes a formal scientific error and is therefore inadmissible.

The reductionist perspective also fails to account for the depth and breadth of human subjectivity. Consciousness, as a phenomenon experienced by the subject, resists reduction to mere neuro-physical processes. It exists at the intersection of material reality and symbolic meaning, intertwined with language, culture, and individual development. This complex interplay points to the necessity of a multidimensional approach—one that transcends strict materialism while remaining grounded in empirical evidence.

Reflecting on the mind–body debate, it becomes clear that reductive explanations cannot capture the essence of human experience. The psyche, understood etymologically and mythologically as a life-giving force, encompasses far more than the functions of the brain. It connects to creativity, imagination, and the symbolic realm, all of which defy simple mechanistic explanations.

The development of consciousness in evolutionary terms suggests a gradual emergence of self-awareness, mirrored in the ontogenetic progression of the young child. This process, as described by Lacan and others, involves separation, identification, and the negotiation of symbolic meaning. Such transitions are fraught with challenges, as evidenced by the vulnerabilities inherent in psychotic disorders and other psychopathologies.

Despite the rise of neuroscience and its contributions to understanding the brain's mechanisms, the existential and phenomenological dimensions of human experience remain elusive. To dismiss these aspects as irrelevant or secondary is to overlook what makes us uniquely human. Consciousness, desire, and imagination are not reducible to mere neuronal activity; they are deeply rooted in the symbolic structures that shape our lives.

In conclusion, the interplay between body and mind, material and symbolic, continues to challenge our understanding. By acknowledging the limitations of reductionist approaches and embracing interdisciplinary collaboration, we can strive for a more comprehensive understanding of the psyche—a concept as rich and multifaceted as humanity itself.

12

SKETCH OF AN ALTERNATIVE

The lack of a physical substrate for psychosis challenges the reductionist biological paradigm prevalent in modern psychiatry. While neuroleptics play a supportive role, particularly in creating stability, they cannot replace the therapeutic necessity of human connection, proximity, and a listening ear. The alternative model outlined here advocates for a holistic integration of physical and psychological treatments, ensuring that the subject remains central to the therapeutic process.

Alternative treatment for people with psychosis does not mean setting aside psychopharmaceuticals and other physical interventions, but rather creating more space for the therapist's speaking and listening. Psychosis also has a story. This means that the therapist must have, or develop, a sensitivity to this narrative. It often involves following one's own psychotherapeutic path and being open to the possibility of encountering one's own psychotic symptoms.

Even though serious psychiatric patients (such as those with borderline conditions or psychosis) struggle with symbolizing themselves and their surroundings, this does not mean that we, as therapists, should turn our backs on them and simply medicate them. No human being can endure loneliness without contact with others. To that end, we therapists must make every effort to learn to understand psychiatric patients or, at the very least, to listen to them. This requires a different attitude than what is generally assumed in psychiatry.

Just because there is no known substrate for the mind, let alone for most psychiatric disorders, does not mean that treatment is impossible. Since the brain is now understood as a plastic organ that undergoes changes when

DOI: 10.4324/9781003675389-17

influenced externally, psychotherapy has gained more credibility, even in an era of predominantly materialistic thinking in psychiatry. There are additional reasons to view psychotherapy as a meaningful treatment approach, but I will not address them here. Somatic treatments can also be effective in psychiatric disorders, particularly psychotropic drugs that have the ability to calm or stimulate patients. Examples include antidepressants and neuroleptics.

Since no substrate for psychosis has been identified, no causal treatment is possible. This is not uncommon in medicine, but in psychiatry, the gap between somatic causes and treatment is particularly striking. The psychotropic drugs used to treat psychoses do not target any underlying etiology. This contrasts sharply with the beliefs held by many professionals, especially within the pharmaceutical industry. Occasionally, psychotic patients also express a hopeful expectation of these treatments, but such instances are rare. This optimism represents a relatively new phenomenon in psychiatry, contrasting with the skepticism that characterized the anti-psychiatry movement during my training as a psychiatrist.

This is not to suggest that psychotropic drugs, particularly neuroleptics, have no effect. On the contrary, antipsychotic drugs are often sedating, though some more so than others. However, it is unlikely that they directly target the core of psychosis, primarily because such a target does not exist. It is an empirical observation that hallucinations are more sensitive to antipsychotics than delusions, likely due to the sedative properties of these drugs. Delusions, on the other hand, rarely disappear with neuroleptic use. While patients may become less communicative about their inner world under the influence of these drugs, closer examination often reveals that their paranoid core beliefs remain intact.

Psychotic patients are frequently confronted with the side effects of antipsychotic medications, which can include stiff limbs, movement restlessness, excessive salivation, jaw locking, weight gain, and even sudden death. These adverse effects are deeply unpleasant and often lead patients to discontinue their medication.

I am not suggesting that neuroleptics should never be used, but their application must be prudent and critical. Medication should be prescribed in consultation with the patient, in limited doses, and certainly not continued rigorously until all psychotic symptoms disappear. Such an approach benefits no one, least of all the patient.

At times, it seems as if drug treatment is the only option for psychosis, with all other interventions deemed secondary. I strongly oppose this perspective. Contact with individuals experiencing psychosis is crucial, even when they appear withdrawn into their autistic cocoon (Koehler et al., 2013; Hinshelwood & Skogstad, 2000). Many patients are eager to talk about their psychotic ideas and experiences, but practitioners often lack the time to listen, or they dismiss these narratives as mere evidence of illness. Today's psychiatrists are often preoccupied with their computers or meetings, driven by the compulsive regulatory demands of governments and insurance companies. Additionally, nursing staff are frequently intimidated by the strange and sometimes paroxysmal behaviors of patients, leading them to withdraw into the safety of the nursing station.

However, there are also nurses who approach psychotic patients with natural intuition and understanding, even without formal training in psychopathology. These nurses engage with patients in a straightforward, humane manner, listening attentively and responding without resorting to rigid disciplinary tactics. Witnessing this kind of care is deeply rewarding.

It is also essential to engage psychotic patients in meaningful activities that help them feel they have a place in society. Many of us are familiar with the phenomenon where even the most sedated and introverted patient becomes actively involved in a crisis. At Delta Hospital in Poortugaal (near Rotterdam), where I trained as an assistant, the nearby Oude Maas overflowed at one point, threatening the hospital grounds. Patients who usually spent their days smoking or lying in bed sprang into action, filling sandbags to reinforce the dike.

Since psychosis lacks a defined substrate, there is no causal somatic treatment available. Psychotropic drugs, while widely used, do not address the root cause of psychosis. Nonetheless, they often provide sedation, which may suppress hallucinations. However, there is no evidence to suggest a causal effect on hallucinations or delusions. Delusions are particularly resistant to neuroleptics. While these medications may reduce the intensity of delusions by sedating the patient, the paranoid core beliefs usually persist.

I do not advocate abandoning neuroleptics entirely but emphasize their cautious use in collaboration with the patient. High doses intended to eliminate symptoms without considering the patient's overall structure often result in fatigue, neurological complications, and other physical and psychological discomforts. It takes more than medication to support individuals with psychosis effectively.

What concerns me most is the increasing loneliness of patients with psychosis. Greater efforts to engage with these individuals through conversation and connection are urgently needed in psychiatry. Unfortunately, many practitioners rely on protocols and mechanistic approaches, further isolating their patients. Establishing meaningful contact requires insight into the patient's personality structure. The strangeness in psychotic individuals is often misunderstood and dismissed with a superficial diagnosis that reassures the practitioner but alienates the patient. True connection demands that therapists confront the strangeness within themselves, including their own experiences of emptiness—an endeavor many find daunting.

Mental health workers must learn to communicate with psychotic patients without imposing the medical framework of diagnosis and drug treatment. In truth, we know relatively little about psychosis, and we stand to learn much from experiential experts. By listening to psychotic individuals, we can help mitigate their profound loneliness.

In this book, we have sought to present an alternative vision of psychiatry, one grounded in French structuralism, which offers the promise of a new approach to treating psychosis. For a long time, I have been frustrated by psychiatry's drift toward a mechanistic praxis. In embracing and canonizing objectivism, psychiatry has crushed the subjective, creating a rigid framework that is now cracking at its seams.

My introduction to structuralism was liberating. Lacan and Foucault pointed the way, and as I reflect on this intellectual journey, I am drawn back to Ferdinand de Saussure, whose ideas inspired the structuralists. Saussure's distinction between denotation and connotation revolutionized thought, replacing rigid denotative thinking with connotative discourse that fosters creativity and freedom of thought. This distinction, and the gap between word and thing, has been a recurring theme in this work, cutting across various levels of psychiatry. Psychiatry, it seems, has become entrenched in denotative thinking, clinging to it in a futile attempt to better grasp the subject. This endeavor, however, appears doomed to fail.

Saussure and the structuralists liberated Western thought from its autistic tendencies. It is now psychiatry's turn.

The liberation of psychiatry from its mechanistic and denotative straitjacket requires a fundamental shift in perspective. This is not merely a theoretical or academic exercise but a practical necessity for improving the treatment and understanding of psychosis. Structuralism offers a framework that embraces the complexity of the human experience, acknowledging the interplay between language, culture, and subjective meaning. In this approach, patients are no longer reduced to symptoms or diagnostic labels but are understood as individuals embedded in a rich tapestry of symbolic and personal contexts.

One of the central challenges in psychiatry is addressing the subjectivity of psychosis without losing sight of its profound strangeness. Psychotic experiences often defy conventional logic and can appear impenetrable to those who are not experiencing them. Yet these experiences are deeply meaningful to the individuals who live through them. A structuralist perspective encourages us to see these narratives as part of a broader dialogue between the individual and the symbolic order in which they exist. This approach does not dismiss psychotic expressions as mere pathology but seeks to understand their significance within the patient's unique worldview.

For practitioners, this means stepping away from the safety of rigid protocols and embracing the uncertainty inherent in working with psychosis. It requires a willingness to listen without judgment and to engage with the patient as a whole person rather than as a collection of symptoms. This is not an easy task, as it demands both intellectual flexibility and emotional courage. However, it is essential if we are to move beyond the limitations of current psychiatric practice.

The role of language in psychosis is particularly noteworthy. Lacan's insights into the relationship between language and the unconscious provide valuable tools for understanding how psychotic individuals navigate their inner and outer worlds. In psychosis, the symbolic structures that typically mediate our experiences of reality can become fragmented or distorted, leading to profound disruptions in perception and meaning. By engaging with the patient's language and exploring the underlying structures of their experiences, therapists can begin to piece together the threads of a shared understanding.

This process of engagement is not merely about decoding symptoms or resolving delusions; it is about building a bridge between the patient's subjective reality and the shared symbolic order. Such a bridge offers the possibility of connection, not only for the patient but also for the therapist, who must confront their own assumptions and biases in the process.

Structuralism also challenges the reductionist tendencies of contemporary psychiatry by emphasizing the role of context and relationality in mental health. The experiences of psychosis cannot be fully understood in isolation from the social, cultural, and linguistic frameworks that shape them. This broader perspective opens up new possibilities for intervention, from community-based approaches to more inclusive and dialogical forms of therapy.

Moreover, structuralism calls into question the dominance of biological reductionism in psychiatry. While neuroscience has provided valuable insights into the brain's functioning, it has also contributed to a narrow focus on the brain as the sole determinant of mental health. This perspective risks obscuring the richness and diversity of human experience, reducing complex phenomena to mere biochemical processes. A structuralist approach reintroduces the human dimension, reminding us that mental health is not just about brain chemistry but also about meaning, relationships, and the symbolic structures that define our existence.

In practice, this means creating spaces where psychotic individuals can express themselves freely and be met with genuine curiosity and respect. It means fostering environments that prioritize connection over control, where the focus is not solely on symptom management but on supporting the individual's journey toward a more integrated sense of self. Such an approach is not only more humane but also more effective in addressing the root causes of suffering.

The future of psychiatry lies in its ability to adapt and evolve, embracing new ideas while remaining grounded in the lived realities of its patients. Structuralism offers a pathway forward, one that honors the complexity of the human experience and recognizes the transformative power of language and meaning. By adopting this perspective, psychiatry can move beyond its current limitations and become a more compassionate and effective discipline.

In conclusion, the journey from denotative to connotative thinking is not just an intellectual shift; it is a moral imperative. Psychiatry's reliance on rigid frameworks and mechanistic models has left many patients feeling alienated and misunderstood. Structuralism offers an alternative that prioritizes dialogue, connection, and the richness of subjective experience. It invites us to see patients not as problems to be solved but as individuals with stories to tell and worlds to share. This shift requires courage, creativity, and a willingness to embrace uncertainty—but the rewards, both for patients and practitioners, are profound.

It is time for psychiatry to embrace this liberation and rediscover the humanity at its core.

PART 5

The Creative Power of Nothingness

Introduction

In this part, I turn to some philosophers to explore their treatment of nothingness. Do they substantiate nihilism, or are there thinkers who view nothingness as a category that inspires something new, as a creative moment? While the previous chapters offered a vision and critique of contemporary psychiatry, this chapter aims to show that the *zero degree* is not only a vital event for the individual human condition but also applies to cultural and social matters, including medical care such as psychiatry. Good care depends on a broad understanding of its object: the human being. The subject is a flawed being, and so forth.

DOI: 10.4324/9781003675389-18

13

FRIEDRICH NIETZSCHE AND DEGREE ZERO OF MORALITY

Nietzsche was not the first philosopher to explore the concept of nothingness, but his work profoundly shaped its contemporary understanding. From Parmenides to Kant, Hegel, and Heidegger, the philosophical lineage of nothingness has been well-documented. Nietzsche, however, highlighted its implications for morality, rejecting conventional structures such as God, religion, and science. His philosophy underscores the groundlessness of thought, paving the way for creative reimaginings of existence.

One can rightly say that "*Zur Genealogie der Moral. Eine Streitschrift*" (On the Genealogy of Moral: A Polemic) is Nietzsche's most controversial book (Nietzsche, 1887). Earlier he had already fulminated against the religions that had enslaved man to morality and with that he had sowed the wind of resentment to revolt against the masters, but in this book—which is not for nothing *Eine Streitschrift* has been mentioned—he analyzes to the bone where morality comes from. He has condensed his entire philosophy as a "counterthinker" into this book. He wrote it in one breath. After that, only a firm statement had to be made in his "Antichrist" (Nietzsche, 1888).

Nietzsche was also an origin seeker and to arrive at that starting point he first had to topple a number of sacred houses: religion, morality, and science.

Although Freud does not often refer to Nietzsche, he does show that he has read him and that he has at least followed him in his aversion to the scientificization of historiography, as is apparent from "Totem and Taboo" and "The Man Moses and Monotheism," in which he gives free rein to fiction. In these texts he tells of the murder of the primeval father and the murder of Moses by the Jewish people and relates this to the Oedipus

DOI: 10.4324/9781003675389-19

complex. Freud distills the proof of this from what his patients tell him in the consulting room. The history of mankind has settled in their unconscious (de Kroon & Houppermans, in print). Of course he had no obvious evidence for this, but from the stories of his patients, he concluded that there was a strong similarity in both the content and the structure of their verbal expressions.

Nietzsche is repeatedly portrayed as a nihilist *pur sang*, because he declared God dead, and he rebelled against the religion, morality, and science with which he presented himself as a naturalistic thinker. The opposite is true. He just wanted to expose and tear down the false certainties Western man was saddled with in order to show that only one indisputable truth remained. With his idea of "Der Wille zur Macht."[1] a quote may clarify that: "*Was bedeutet Nihilismus?—Dass die oberste Werte sich entwerden. Es fehlt das Ziel. Es fehlt die Antwort auf das 'Wozu?'.*"[2] (Nietzsche, 1887). History has no purpose, only an eternal repetition of the same thing.

With regard to the prevailing certainties, Nietzsche can rightly be called a nihilist, but by means of an *Umwertung aller Werte*,[3] he nevertheless arrives at something that provides a certain foundation. Nietzsche could also be regarded as a chronicler of his time, when belief in values and meaning was on the wane. What remained was a frenzied search for the truth that people thought they would find in physical reality. That was also the time of the rise of natural science, in which people had almost infinite confidence. Initially, Nietzsche flirted here and there with natural science but in the course of time distanced himself from it as an obstacle to the truth of life. Man's being is based on nothing. It is *Der Wille zur Macht* (The Will to Power) that keeps people going. There is no other motive (Nietzsche, 1886, 2017).

Nietzsche opposes the nihilism of his time and wants to install in its place a vitalism that does justice to the true nature of man. That is an aspect of *Der Wille zur Macht*, which has often been the cause of misunderstandings. The will to power in Nietzsche is not a desire for power from one person over another or an expression of lust for power, but rather a principle of life, an expression of vitality. The power of the *Übermensch* is expressed in his positioning in life at the risk of his own life. This person is not cowardly and does not allow himself to be included in the mob of slaves who huddle together and confuse themselves with edifying stories and moral fairy tales. The slave is cowardly and flees from death and uses his morals as a weapon against the master. He is jealous of his master. His morals are submissive, masochistic, and cowardly, but the slaves are many and are up against a small minority. The slaves know that in the long run the masters will also have to recognize and adopt the slave morality. Democracy is born.

The master is characterized by force: "A quantum force is an equal quantum of drive, will, activity—or rather, it is nothing but this very drive, will, being active itself" (Nietzsche, 1887). It remains uncertain here what quality Nietzsche ascribes to the "drive." I suspect that Freud read this passage with Nietzsche and does not consider the drive purely naturalistic but situates the drive between soma and psyche (Freud, 1933).

Nietzsche goes further and attributes the decline of power to language or the petrified interpretation that an impulse has become a "subject," a substrate. But according to him, there is no such substrate behind the purpose of a quantum force. The naturalists, too, commit this error by saying, "The force moves, the force causes" (Nietzsche, 1887, p. 37).

Der Wille zur Macht is not a pamphlet with an apodictic position but a philosophy of life that Nietzsche defends fervently throughout his oeuvre. When *der Wille zur Macht*, which is an essential part of life, has to make way for slave morality, arguments are used to justify this shift in morality. One reasoning is to place the truth with God, and the other is to incorporate a conception that contains an alternative truth and leads to science. When the balance of power changes, morality also changes. Power is a relational matter and not something substantial that can be referred to as a fixed standard. That is also the reason why power relations change so often and morality keeps pace with it.

Notes

1 Nietzsche(1901), The will to power. This was his last project that did not come to a publication. In the end he split it into Götterdämerung and the Antichrist.
2 "What does nihilism mean?—That the supreme values will disintegrate. The goal is missing. The answer to the 'Why?' is missing."
3 "Revaluation of all values."

14

INTERLUDE

Fable

A brief interlude presents a fictional narrative that illustrates key themes of the book, including the transformative potential of nothingness and its role in creativity and human experience.

Just a Brainwave

When God was alive he was alone. Nothing around him and he wondered what he could do to dispel the boredom. Nothing lasted long and nothing ever happened. There was no one who could listen to everything that was going on inside him, no one to whom he could tell his dreams and fantasies. The nothing gave no answer and gave no sign of life at all.

God thought something must come instead of nothing, "Not just anything, but something good, something that matches the most perfect fantasy I have." He thought for a long time because you don't just create something like that. It had to be something that wouldn't disappoint him and that he wouldn't regret later. After a very long time of thinking he decided to create something and in one week he would actually work it out and he wanted to start the next Monday. However, on Monday morning he suddenly began to doubt: "Would it be good to make something? Isn't it better to just leave it at nothing? Wouldn't it be better to just let his fantasy go?" He couldn't consult anyone for a second opinion. All alone he had to make this decision. That same day he took the plunge and decided to take a chance. And so it happened on that memorable Monday. First the light, then the earth, then life, and finally the word, or had he just

DOI: 10.4324/9781003675389-20

begun with that? Since then, this day has also been called splitting Monday because a distinction was made between nothing and something.

Now after so many billions of years of ever advancing developments in which the stars and planets came into being, the light was separated from the darkness and life arose as on planet earth, it is time to take stock. And there we stand and look around us and tell each other our history but shrink from looking into the future, because it is obscured to us humans. There is no one who can say anything about that, but we are holding our breath because the signs are not favorable. We cannot turn back the clock and must move on; there's no turning back.

In the meantime, a great deal has emerged that we embrace with enthusiasm but whose weight also weighs on us. We are in danger of succumbing to the increasing weight. Breathing becomes more and more difficult, and we feel death approaching. Who or what can save us? We realize that we have to solve it ourselves, because in the course of time we have killed God. The creator of the something might have been able to turn the tide, but he is dead. There are those who deny that there was murder but say that God Himself took his own life as a result of severe depression related to his disappointment at his creation. We won't know, but the fact is, we're on our own. The father who could have saved us is dead. There we are.

Creation has always had a positive connotation. When an artist has completed a work, he is usually relieved and in some cases also satisfied. It is usually the readers and museum visitors who admire a work of art. Making something is usually well regarded. That is in stark contrast to the nothingness that has a bad reputation. The nihilism that embraces nothingness has always had a bad odor in the history of Western culture. When I say "I don't believe in anything" people look at me strangely and usually with pity. "Poor man" they think. "It would be better for him if he had something to hold on to." Postmodern man has a hard time; he has nothing to hold on to, he believes in nothing. Not in God, not in the Other, he even doubts the existence of matter. Perhaps existence is a fiction. He must be careful not to become psychotic.

15

MARTIN HEIDEGGER AND NOTHINGNESS

For Heidegger, nothingness is a metaphysical concept with profound existential implications. It is not an entity with extension but a force that shapes being itself. Heidegger describes how nothingness provokes fear (horror vacui), compelling humans to fill the void through speech. Language, for Heidegger, becomes both a means of confronting and transcending this existential emptiness.

Heidegger was an admirer of Nietzsche and continued the exploration of nothingness to further develop this theme. As a thinker of *Being*, it shows both courage and insight to also confront *non-being*.

For Heidegger, nothingness is a reality to which humans intuitively resist, a resistance that is expressed in language. In his *Der Satz vom Grund* (*The Principle of Ground*, 1956, 1974), Heidegger takes the position that there is no ultimate foundation for the words we use to signify reality. This applies not only to morality but, in fact, to everything we as human beings encounter and attempt to articulate. There is no basis for the word. We humans must learn to live with that.

Heidegger's Critique of Nietzsche and the Question of Nothingness

Heidegger dared to criticize Nietzsche. In his *Was ist Metaphysik?* (*What is Metaphysics?*), he reproaches Nietzsche for remaining trapped in metaphysics when elaborating the essence of nothingness, even though Nietzsche aimed to overcome it. Let us follow Heidegger's reasoning (Heidegger, 1929). When we trace the concept of nothingness, it is not an absolute

DOI: 10.4324/9781003675389-21

nothingness, for if it were, there would be no question of anything at all. Science, which is preeminently concerned with being, raises the question of nothingness when delineating its own object. This duality between something and nothing is an essential feature of science. Naturally, this leads to the metaphysical question of nothingness.

How is it possible to experience nothingness within the realm of being? A finite being cannot comprehend the entirety of being but can situate itself within the whole of being. There appears to be a boundary, veiled by nothingness. Confronting nothingness evokes fear. This fear, distinct from anxiety, is indefinable; it offers no foothold. Fundamentally, this fear relates to death, a terror against which humanity has devised countless strategies of avoidance. In the face of nothingness, stripped of language or certainty, a person experiences only the void of existence. Humanity takes a stance toward being, distancing itself from it, transcending it. Nothingness is not a thing, nor the opposite of being. Humanity does not entirely coincide with being; rather, it takes a position relative to being. It exists—it stands outside itself. The awareness of finitude instills fear, leading humanity to turn away from nothingness. Heidegger asserts that humanity "destroys" nothingness. Our aversion to nothingness has influenced language itself, creating negations: "I'm not going," "I don't know," "I don't want that," and so on. The individual who inquires into nothingness inevitably engages in metaphysics.

This raises the question: Do we enter the world as blank slates? From birth, we adopt the customs and achievements of our environment, first from parents or caregivers and later from those around us. We absorb the culture into which we are "thrown" with a natural eagerness. Heidegger's concept of "thrownness" (*Geworfenheit*) aptly captures this, as no choice is involved at the beginning of life; free will is a capacity that emerges only later, when we are equipped to exercise it. It is the desire of others—particularly our parents—that brings us into existence. Later, in the course of development, autonomy arises, manifesting as (self-)consciousness and free will. However, complete independence from the Other is an illusion. Even a thinker as radically individualistic as Nietzsche, a master of the *Umwertung aller Werte* (*revaluation of all values*), never entirely detached himself from morality. Instead, he sought to create a new morality based on nothing.

Existence is not autogenous from the outset. We begin with nothing, gradually filled by influences from outside—by the Other. The word "exist" itself reflects this: we exist from the outside, shaped by ingredients supplied by the Other. Lacan's term "extimate" beings (*extimité*) aptly describes us (Lacan, 1966).

Life is contingent in every respect. Against the abyss of this contingency, humanity arms itself with ideologies, religion, and grand narratives. In the (post-)modern era, having discarded these protective strategies, we face the yawning chasm of nothingness. The grand narratives have been unmasked by science—not only as false but also as instruments of control. Yet science, a relatively young grand narrative, fails to recognize that it too serves as a way to soothe our fear of nothingness. Like religion and ideology, it seeks to fill the void. The question remains: How long will this new illusion last?

Nothingness continues to haunt humanity. Born from nothingness, we carry it with us throughout life, manifesting as the fear of death—the ultimate nothingness.

Yet nothingness also has its positive aspects. Humanity cannot tolerate nothingness; we strive to nullify it, to fill it with something. We row against the current to overcome the death drive and avoid its pull (Moyaert, 2015). One might even say that we exist by the grace of nothingness.

Sartre suggests that being and nothingness form an inseparable pair, connected by the Logos. The famous soliloquy from *Hamlet*, "To be or not to be," is thus paradoxical. There is no true contradiction; being and not being belong together, like the inhalation and exhalation of breath. It is tempting to think of filling the gap of being with matter or objects, but in practice, this proves insufficient. Indeed, it often leads to a sense of disgust, as seen in addiction. For Lacan, the highest way to meet desire is through sublimation. Symbolization, while imperfect, transforms desire into something meaningful. The word itself is insufficient to satisfy desire; it is precisely the inadequacy of language that evokes new desires. Words always leave a gap in being (Lacan, 1966).

Does nothingness exist at all, or is it merely a product of language (*ens rationalis et orationis*)? Darkness, for example, is not the nothingness of light but its negation—a *nihil privativum* (Kant, 1781–1787). Hegel, however, posits the existence of a pure nothingness, a complete emptiness that is not a contradiction of anything. This is an aimless negation, something inexpressible. While negation always presupposes an object, Hegel argues for a nothingness without object. For him, pure nothingness justifies an absolute principle, grounded in religion and the genealogy of the humanities. He even claims, "Pure being and pure nothing are thus the same" (Hegel, 1807). Whether nothingness is an absolute principle or a product of symbolization, the Hegelian dialectic holds when being and nothingness converge. Is this a matter of metaphysics? Does it not become paradoxical when Hegel claims that being and nothingness are one and the same?

Has being always existed, with nothingness intermingling with it until consciousness emerged? Or did being itself arise (was created?) out of nothing? I am inclined to believe that being has a certain permanence, that it is eternal. The symbolic, on the other hand, seems to have emerged from nothingness. Or should we assume that there was indeed a creation?

The question of whether being arose from nothing or has always existed is central to both metaphysical inquiry and the human condition. If being is eternal, it suggests a kind of permanence that grounds existence, providing a foundation for the symbolic and material realities we inhabit. Yet, if being itself emerged from nothing, it implies a fundamental contingency that colors our understanding of life, identity, and purpose. Either way, the interplay between being and nothingness remains inescapable.

In this context, the notion of creation becomes a key point of contention. For those who adhere to religious or spiritual frameworks, creation is an intentional act—a moment when something was brought forth from nothing by a divine will or cosmic principle. Conversely, secular interpretations often lean toward an emergent perspective, where being arises from chaos or randomness without a guiding hand. Both perspectives, however, wrestle with the same fundamental dilemma: how to account for the transition from non-being to being.

This tension is reflected in existentialist thought. Sartre's claim that existence precedes essence rejects the idea of a predetermined purpose or design, placing the burden of meaning squarely on the individual. For Sartre, human existence is marked by radical freedom, but this freedom is accompanied by the weight of nothingness—the absence of inherent meaning or purpose. It is within this void that individuals must forge their own values, a task both liberating and burdensome.

Heidegger, by contrast, sees nothingness as a horizon against which being reveals itself. For him, the experience of nothingness is not merely a philosophical abstraction but an essential aspect of human existence. It is in moments of profound anxiety—when all familiar certainties fall away—that the individual confronts the groundlessness of being. This encounter with nothingness is not a negation of life but a precondition for authentic existence. By facing the void, we are compelled to take responsibility for our own being and to engage more deeply with the world.

Lacan extends this inquiry into the realm of psychoanalysis, where the symbolic order plays a central role in mediating the relationship between being and nothingness. For Lacan, the subject is inherently split, caught between the imaginary and the symbolic, with nothingness functioning as a persistent lack that drives desire. This lack is not a flaw to be remedied but an integral aspect of human subjectivity. It is the gap between what we are and what we aspire to be that propels us forward, compelling us to create, to symbolize, and to seek meaning.

In this sense, nothingness is not merely an absence; it is a productive force. It inspires art, science, and philosophy, pushing humanity to transcend its limitations and engage with the unknown. Yet this same nothingness also evokes fear and anxiety, as it reminds us of our finitude and the ultimate unknowability of existence. The duality of nothingness—as both a source of creativity and a reminder of mortality—lies at the heart of the human condition.

The modern era, characterized by the decline of religious and ideological certainties, has brought this duality into sharper focus. Without the grand narratives that once provided a sense of purpose and stability, we are left to confront the void directly. Science, while offering powerful tools for understanding the material world, cannot fully address the existential questions that arise in the face of nothingness. Its explanatory frameworks often fall short when it comes to the intangible aspects of human experience—meaning, love, death, and the sublime.

This leaves us with the challenge of living meaningfully in a world that offers no guarantees. How can we navigate the tension between being and nothingness without succumbing to despair or nihilism? The answer, perhaps, lies in embracing the paradox itself. By acknowledging the interplay between presence and absence, fullness and void, we can begin to see nothingness not as a threat but as an opportunity—a space for growth, transformation, and renewal.

In art and literature, this paradox is often explored with profound insight. The act of creation, whether through painting, writing, or music, is a testament to humanity's ability to wrest something from nothing. Each work of art is a defiance of the void, a declaration that existence matters, even if its ultimate purpose remains elusive. Similarly, philosophical and scientific pursuits reflect a relentless drive to make sense of the unknown, to illuminate the darkness with the light of understanding.

In conclusion, the relationship between being and nothingness is not one to be resolved but one to be lived. It is a dynamic interplay that shapes every aspect of our existence, from our deepest fears to our greatest aspirations. Whether framed in metaphysical, existential, or psychoanalytic terms, this tension invites us to confront the fundamental questions of life with courage and creativity. In doing so, we affirm our place in the cosmos—not as passive observers but as active participants in the ongoing dance of being and nothingness.

The interplay between being and nothingness not only shapes individual existence but also collective human endeavors. Societies, much like individuals, are defined by their response to the void. Throughout history, civilizations have constructed intricate systems of belief, culture, and governance to contend with the underlying anxiety of nothingness. These frameworks have served as shields against the abyss, offering coherence and purpose to communal life.

Religious narratives, for example, provide not only cosmological explanations but also existential solace. By positing a divine order or ultimate purpose, they fill the void with meaning, creating a sense of continuity that transcends individual mortality. Even as secularism has gained prominence, the echoes of these narratives persist in our collective imagination, shaping how we understand life and death, creation and destruction.

Science, as a modern grand narrative, has taken on a similar role. By unveiling the mechanics of the universe and uncovering the laws of nature, science promises a kind of certainty in the face of uncertainty. Yet, as Heidegger points out, this promise is ultimately limited. Science can explain *how* things work but often falters when addressing the deeper *why*. The more we understand the mechanisms of existence, the more apparent the void becomes. Science, for all its achievements, cannot escape the fundamental contingency of being.

Art, on the other hand, thrives on this tension. Artists engage directly with the void, transforming it into a space of creation. Where science seeks to map and define, art explores and evokes. The most profound works of art are those that confront the paradox of being and nothingness head-on, offering not solutions but experiences that resonate with the complexity of existence. In this way, art becomes a bridge between the tangible and the ineffable, a testament to humanity's capacity to live meaningfully within the void.

Philosophy, too, occupies a unique space in this dialogue. From Hegel's dialectic to Sartre's existentialism, philosophical inquiry grapples with the fundamental questions of being and nothingness, seeking not to resolve them but to articulate their significance. Heidegger's emphasis on the experience of being-toward-death, for instance, challenges us to confront our finitude without retreating into denial or despair. This confrontation, far from negating life, enhances it by grounding us in the present and sharpening our awareness of what it means to exist.

In the postmodern era, where grand narratives have been deconstructed and skepticism reigns supreme, the void looms larger than ever. Without the unifying myths of the past, we are left to navigate a fragmented world, where meaning is contingent and truth is plural. This condition, while disorienting, also offers unprecedented freedom. Freed from the constraints of absolute certainties, we have the opportunity to redefine what it means to be human.

However, this freedom is not without its challenges. The absence of universal truths can lead to a sense of alienation, as individuals struggle to find their place in a world that seems increasingly indifferent. This alienation is compounded by the rapid pace of technological change, which often amplifies feelings of disconnection and transience. In such a context, the question of nothingness becomes more urgent than ever: How do we fill the void in a way that is authentic and sustainable?

One possible answer lies in rethinking our relationship with the void itself. Rather than viewing nothingness as a deficiency to be overcome, we can embrace it as a space of possibility. As Lacan suggests, desire arises precisely from the gap between what is and what could be. This gap, far from being a source of despair, can become a wellspring of creativity and transformation. By engaging with the void—through art, philosophy, relationships, and action—we can forge new paths that honor the complexity and ambiguity of existence.

This approach requires a shift in perspective, one that prioritizes process over outcome and experience over certainty. It invites us to see life not as a problem to be solved but as a mystery to be lived. In this view, the interplay of being and nothingness is not a contradiction to be resolved but a dynamic tension that animates everything we do. It is the source of our fears and aspirations, our failures and triumphs, and our despair and hope.

As we face the challenges of the modern world—from ecological crises to social fragmentation—we must draw on this deeper understanding of being and nothingness. The solutions we seek will not come from denying the void or clinging to outdated certainties but from engaging with the complexity of our situation in all its fullness. By embracing the paradox of existence, we can find new ways to live, create, and connect—ways that acknowledge both the fragility and resilience of the human spirit.

In the end, the question of nothingness is inseparable from the question of what it means to be alive. It is a question that defies easy answers, demanding instead a lifelong engagement with the mysteries of existence. As Heidegger, Sartre, Lacan, and others have shown, this engagement is not a burden but an opportunity—a chance to explore the depths of being and to shape a life that is both meaningful and true.

The Paradox of Creation and Destruction

The relationship between being and nothingness also reveals an inherent paradox in creation itself. To create something is to bring it into existence, but this act of creation simultaneously defines the boundaries of what it is not. Every creation casts a shadow of absence. In this way, creation and destruction are inextricably linked, as each new existence displaces what was previously present or potential. This interplay shapes not only our physical world but also our intellectual, emotional, and cultural landscapes.

Nietzsche captures this paradox in his concept of the *Umwertung aller Werte* (*revaluation of all values*), where the destruction of old values is a precondition for the emergence of new ones. This dynamic is not limited to morality but applies to all domains of human existence. Science, art, philosophy, and even individual identity evolve through cycles of creation and dissolution. Each act of innovation or transformation entails the loss of something that once was, leaving a void in its wake—a void that invites further creation.

In this light, nothingness is not simply the absence of being but an active and generative force. It challenges us to confront the limits of our understanding, pushing us to imagine and articulate what lies beyond. Heidegger's notion of *Gelassenheit* (*releasement*) offers a way of engaging with this dynamic. By letting go of our need for control and certainty, we can approach being and nothingness with openness and receptivity, allowing them to unfold in their fullness.

The Weight of Freedom

One of the greatest challenges posed by the modern encounter with nothingness is the burden of freedom. As Sartre famously argued, the absence of predetermined meaning forces individuals to take responsibility for their own existence. This freedom, while empowering, is also a source of profound anxiety. Without external certainties to guide us, we must confront the weight of our choices and the finitude of our lives.

This existential burden often leads to what Kierkegaard called "the sickness unto death"—a despair born from the realization that we are free yet finite, capable of infinite possibilities but constrained by the limits of our mortality. To navigate this tension, we must find ways to embrace our freedom without being overwhelmed by its implications. For many, this involves constructing personal narratives or frameworks of meaning that provide a sense of coherence and direction, even in the absence of universal truths.

At the collective level, this freedom also raises questions about how societies can function without shared metaphysical foundations. In the absence of grand narratives, how do we build systems of ethics, governance, and culture that respect individual autonomy while fostering solidarity and mutual care? This challenge is particularly acute in a globalized and pluralistic world, where diverse perspectives and values coexist in often uneasy tension.

The Role of Art and Imagination

Art provides a vital means of grappling with these questions. Unlike philosophy or science, which seek to explain or categorize, art allows us to inhabit the ambiguity of being and nothingness. Through its capacity to evoke rather than resolve, art creates spaces where contradictions can coexist, where the fullness of existence can be felt without the need for definitive answers.

In this sense, art is both a reflection of and a response to the void. It mirrors our struggles with meaning, mortality, and desire while offering glimpses of beauty, connection, and transcendence. Whether through painting, music, literature, or other forms of expression, art reminds us that the act of creation is itself an affirmation of life—a defiance of nothingness that transforms absence into presence.

Toward a Philosophy of Embrace

If nothingness is an inevitable aspect of existence, how might we learn to live with it, not as an adversary but as an integral part of life? This question invites us to move beyond the binary opposition of being and nothingness, recognizing their interdependence as a dynamic process. Instead of seeking to conquer or escape the void, we might cultivate a philosophy of embrace—one that acknowledges the fragility and uncertainty of existence while celebrating its possibilities.

Such a philosophy would draw on the insights of thinkers like Heidegger, Sartre, and Lacan, as well as the creative energies of art and literature. It would encourage us to see nothingness not as a deficiency but as a source of potential, a space where new meanings and relationships can emerge. By facing the void with courage and creativity, we can transform it from a symbol of despair into a catalyst for growth and renewal.

The Future of Being and Nothingness

As we look to the future, the interplay between being and nothingness will remain central to our understanding of ourselves and our world. Advances in science and technology will undoubtedly reshape the ways we engage with these questions, offering new tools and perspectives for exploring the nature of existence. Yet these developments will also bring new challenges, as the boundaries between reality and simulation, presence and absence, become increasingly blurred.

In the face of these uncertainties, the wisdom of the past can provide valuable guidance. From the metaphysical inquiries of Hegel and Heidegger to the existential reflections of Sartre and Nietzsche, the philosophical tradition offers a rich repertoire of concepts and approaches for navigating the complexities of being and nothingness. By engaging with these ideas in dialogue with contemporary thought, we can continue to deepen our understanding of what it means to exist.

Ultimately, the question of nothingness is not one to be solved but one to be lived. It is a challenge that calls us to embrace the fullness of life, with all its contradictions and uncertainties. By doing so, we affirm our place in the ever-unfolding drama of being, a drama that is shaped as much by what is absent as by what is present.

16

NOTHINGNESS AT JACQUES LACAN

Lacan, both a psychiatrist and psychoanalyst, was deeply influenced by Heidegger's philosophy and merged it with Freud's psychoanalytic theories. For Lacan, language occupies a central role in structuring human experience, acting as a bridge between the Real, Imaginary, and Symbolic. Freud observed linguistic mechanisms in dreams, while Heidegger employed poetic language to illuminate philosophical concepts. Lacan extended these ideas, positing that the Real, Imaginary, and Symbolic are interwoven but irreducible to each other. This triadic framework provides an epistemological foundation for psychoanalysis and offers profound insights into the nature of psychosis.

Jacques Lacan posits that the subject is founded on nothing and resists this emptiness through the use of language. This effort is ultimately in vain, as every spoken word creates a new void. Yet humanity sustains itself through this Sisyphean labor—groundless work through which the subject maintains the illusion of representing or being something. This is why speaking and listening are so crucial in therapy.

Speaking and listening imply one another. When we no longer lend our ears to each other, we abandon them, which is, in essence, inhumane. This is especially true when listening to patients who are difficult to follow, such as psychotics. To develop a therapeutic listening attitude, significant effort and study are required. Knowledge of the subject is indispensable for this.

DOI: 10.4324/9781003675389-22

Psychoanalysis Is "out," and Lacan Has Never Been "in," at Least Not in the Netherlands

As a form of treatment, psychoanalysis has given way to therapies that claim scientific legitimacy through "evidence-based" methodologies. These approaches often claim a monopoly on truth, even if they defer its attainment to the future. In Freudo-Lacanian thought, however, the relationship to truth and truth itself is problematized. Can we know the truth? Is there such a thing as truth? Questions like these hold little traction in today's scientific world. Regardless, reality is approached by humans through language, and humans themselves seem to be its product. Humanity as an effect of speaking. Speaking plays a decisive role in psychoanalysis. Freud repeatedly emphasized this in his early writings, particularly in his magnum opus, *The Interpretation of Dreams*. One of his patients famously described psychoanalysis as a "talking cure," a highly unusual treatment at the time, when many people with psychological problems visited spas or were treated with chloral hydrate.

In *Retour à Freud*, Lacan sought to underscore this aspect of psychoanalysis, emphasizing a return to Freud's texts and, fundamentally, to the word. Lacan even went so far as to state that "the unconscious is structured like a language." Psychology, aspiring to be part of the scientific tradition, is based on empirical facts and focuses on observable behavior, including language. Psychologists listen to patients and attempt to identify where things went wrong logically. However, as Marc De Kesel notes in his *The Münchhausen Paradigm. Why Freud and Lacan Matter*, Lacan's approach offers a radically different view:

> The theory Lacan recognized in Freud's psychoanalysis is clearly not that kind of "psychology." In his oeuvre, Lacan repeatedly opposes the idea that the therapist must—and can—go beyond talk. He takes a radically different view of what "talking" is. Talk is not mere expression; it is also—first and foremost—an act. However, this is not an act that, as Aristotle thought, connects me with being, with essences that are logical, and with the logos that leads to those essences. According to Lacan, talking is primarily a social act. This is a crucial insight, especially for those who want to understand the subject. Talking builds sociality—not merely because language allows me to communicate with others, but because there is no "I" prior to language. It is not the case that an "I" exists first and then uses the tool of language. In this sense, Lacan's theory is profoundly sociological. Language comes first, always preceding the subject. Language makes the subject possible and "produces" it. Talking cannot be reduced to an instrumental tool that I employ; it is,

> more fundamentally, an act that reaffirms, operationalizes, and makes ever more productive the position I have always occupied within, and thanks to language.
>
> *(De Kesel, 2019)*

This observation aligns with the concept of emptiness discussed in this text. Words do not refer to an essence or a fundamental ground of being; they refer only to other words, endlessly deferring meaning. This principle applies equally to the subject itself. The essence of the subject is never fully accessible. Its words drift, seeking anchors, and land on another word, which also floats in ambiguity, and so on. When we, as subjects, search for ourselves, we rely on a tool that exists outside of us: language.

Language has created a rupture with nature, the origin of humanity. Existence is no longer self-evident; it no longer coincides with nature—a fact that biologists often seem reluctant to confront. De Kesel clarifies this rupture:

> Obviously, we are a part of nature, but we do not live from that nature; rather, we live from the rupture with it—a rupture that has the materiality of a sign system, of language. This makes us, as humans, fundamentally cultural beings, with "culture" defined as that which cannot be reduced to "nature" or "natural laws." Lacan fully adopts this axiom, which underlies Lévi-Strauss's structuralist anthropology. In this sense, what we take as our identity has little basis in "nature" and is predominantly a "cultural" construct. This construct arises from the fact that humans exchange signs with one another and interact on that basis—on the foundation of an autonomously functioning sign system—recognizing themselves as who they are.
>
> *(De Kesel, 2019)*

This rupture with nature ensures that the subject—humanity in its speaking state—no longer entirely coincides with itself. The gap between nature and culture generates a void, a space that yearns to be filled. With what? Ideally, with words; at worst, with hedonic trivialities.

This emptiness, this void, is often referred to as humanity's deficiency, the *manque à être* (*lack of being*), which defines desire.

Where science and psychoanalysis diverge is in their respective approaches to desire and knowledge. Science, driven by a desire for knowledge, seeks to map the unknown through further investigation. Psychoanalysis, however, maintains that knowledge is inherently marked by impossibility. Desire exists in both domains, but in psychoanalysis, the desire for knowledge—the desire to fill the gap in being—remains unresolved. This unresolved nature is a fundamental characteristic of desire and the subject.

For centuries, it was assumed that words express being and that the essence of humanity is revealed in language. Lacan, however, challenges this notion. In his work, he emphasizes that the subject is determined symbolically. Humanity, he argues, is a symbolic being, shaped and signified by language. Humanity is a *parlêtre*—a speaking being. This symbolic nature is closely tied to deficiency (Lacan, 1994). Humanity is marked by a lack, a theme familiar from the Christian tradition, particularly in the doctrine of original sin.

In the myth, humanity was once perfect, whole, and without deficiency. Yet, with the Fall, this changed. Adam and Eve's consumption of the fruit of the tree of knowledge expelled them from paradise. Since then, humanity has been mortal, burdened by knowledge, and terrified by the inevitability of death. Christianity offers hope of redemption through Christ, who bore the sins of the world and died for them. Yet, even with the promise of eternal life, humanity remains marked by deficiency—by the necessity of death.

Lacan, while familiar with the Christian myth and influenced by it, opposed the Catholic faith in which he was raised. Still, the influence of religion is evident throughout his work. Themes such as the Law (Moses) and the Name-of-the-Father (from the Lord's Prayer) resonate in his theories. Although these religious influences are fascinating, they will not be explored further here.

The Symbolic and Deficiency

What does the symbolic have to do with deficiency? To understand this, we must recognize that human knowledge resides in the unconscious, which is a byproduct of conscious existence. Like consciousness, the unconscious has a structure: that of language. According to Lacan, "the unconscious is structured like a language" (Lacan, 1966). Language consists of symbols (*signifiers*) that point to representations (*signifieds*). Between these two—the signifier and the signified—there is an inherent gap, an impossibility. A word cannot fully replace the thing it signifies. The word is not the thing itself (Foucault, 1966). This dynamic creates an intrinsic deficiency in language.

Paradoxically, this impossibility is not a disadvantage. On the contrary, it provides protection and allows us to assign meaning to the world and ourselves. The floating nature of language enables creativity in both the arts and sciences. The barrier between word and thing shields us from the overwhelming intrusion of the Real, much like Perseus's shield protected him from the petrifying gaze of Medusa.

17

SLAVOJ ŽIŽEK

Can It Be Less Than Nothing?

Žižek's exploration of nothingness builds on Lacan and Hegel, suggesting that the subject arises from an absence—a foundational void. Desire emerges from this nothingness, traversing the linguistic chain of signifiers to create meaning. However, the word, as a symbol, never fully captures the essence of the thing it represents, perpetuating the subject's longing. Žižek's analysis deepens our understanding of the structural dynamics at play in subject formation and psychosis.

Slavoj Žižek's *magnum opus* revolves around nothingness. Although he draws from Kant, who revived the theme of nothingness from the dust of modern philosophy, Žižek is also a follower of Lacan. Nevertheless, in this work, he consistently engages with the philosophy of Hegel.

To conclude, Žižek's book *Less Than Nothing*, a profound exploration of the power of nothingness, has been a great source of inspiration to me.

When Žižek describes the subject, he draws upon the work of Immanuel Kant and Jacques Lacan. In both thinkers, the subject lacks any anchoring in substance. It has no roots in matter and finds its essence in a negative formula expressed through language.

In his *Critique of Pure Reason*, Kant sees the subject as a shared being—biologically determined by drives on the one hand and as a spirit that orders the perceived world through pure concepts or categories on the other (Kant, 1781, 1788). This view is not fundamentally different from René Descartes, except that for Descartes, the ego is a thinking thing, a *res cogitans*. We cannot avoid acknowledging that it is the subject that thinks; the *I think*. Thus, the subject is a reality, regardless of how we interpret its

DOI: 10.4324/9781003675389-23

nature. Kant considers this *I think* as the "primordial unity of transcendental apperception." For Kant, transcendental apperception is the essence of self-consciousness, existing outside the perception of empiricism. This difficult concept can be understood as a focused mindfulness that enables self-consciousness through the symbolic mirroring of transcendence. Pure perception, by contrast, does not pass through the mind and therefore need not be transcendental. With Lacan, we see that perception takes place within the domain of the Imaginary. When perception is interpreted—through thinking—it belongs to the Symbolic order, where the thinking subject plays a role (Lacan, 1966).

According to Kant, humans have an almost uncontrollable tendency to substantiate what belongs to the domain of reason—a tendency to transform an idea into a thing. This phenomenon is frequently observed in psychiatry, with diagnoses such as autism, ADHD, and schizophrenia being treated as substantive entities. Kant calls this a transcendental illusion (Ratke, 1930). However, he does not attribute this phenomenon to irrationality, wishful thinking, or uncritical intuition but to reason itself. Reason, Kant argues, is divided within itself (Vande Veire, 2015).

Transcendental apperception is an *a priori* condition that precedes all experience and knowledge of objects (Ratke, 1930). When it comes to nothingness, Kantian concepts such as substance, the *a priori*, and transcendental apperception are crucial for understanding the status of nothingness.

Kant criticizes Descartes for equating the *I* with a substantial entity, a *res cogitans*. The same error can occur with the idea of nothingness, reducing it to a thing that is nothing. There is a tendency to substantiate psychoanalytic concepts, such as the transitional object or the *objet petit a*, turning them into objects of illusion. Yet these are not observable entities; they arise from transcendental apperception.

Kant also posits that certain ideas are fixed *a priori*:

> By this I, or he, or the (thing) that thinks, nothing more is represented than a transcendental subject of thought = x, known only by the thoughts which are its predicates and of which we alone can never have any understanding. We therefore revolve in a continuous circle around the subject. ... And further: "The reason for this lies in the fact that we must necessarily ascribe to things *a priori* all the properties which constitute the conditions without which we cannot think them."
>
> *(Kant, 1787, A 346-347/2004, p. 370)*

Žižek, following Lacan, does not adopt Kant's premise. They reject the notion of pure apperception, asserting instead that the subject is based on nothing. Nothingness generates longing—a longing for the Other to fill the subject—but this fulfillment is never complete. There is always something left to desire. The idea of fully completing the subject is an illusion, which we, as neurotics, must learn to tolerate. More constructively, desire is what propels the subject forward.

Nothingness is filled with something that lacks ground or substance—signifiers that refer to something but repeatedly open up the abyss. A word is not a thing but a symbol. We sustain our illusions through symbols, maintaining the illusion that we are a subject, that we have an *I*, that we are someone. This illusion is necessary; without it, we risk falling into a lifeless nihilism.

At the start of the 20th century, Henri Bergson was a highly popular philosopher and even received the Nobel Prize in Literature. In his best-known work, *L'Évolution créatrice*, he explores a wide range of topics, including Darwin's theory of evolution, time as a creative force, and the concept of nothingness (Bergson, 1906). When Bergson asks why there is something rather than nothing, he refrains from offering a definitive answer. However, he demonstrates that humans cannot tolerate nothingness. We must act to destroy the void. This unprovoked action often gives rise to something new, something creative. This applies not only to composers and writers but also to ordinary people who create something in life. Moreover, it applies to every person who comes into the world and takes the revolutionary step of symbolizing—arming themselves against (the fear of) nothingness. Symbolization, or mastering language, allows us to engage with the world and protects us from the overwhelming nature of nothingness and the Real.

Bergson's philosophy centers on humanity's creative capacity. However, it remains unclear whether his *élan vital* is the cause or the result of this process. Is the *élan vital* the origin of humanity's discomfort with nothingness, or is it the intolerance of nothingness that generates the *élan vital*? Perhaps cause and effect are dialectically related. Either way, this drive, as articulated by Bergson, is integral to life and often leads to creative breakthroughs.

This corrected version maintains clarity and preserves the nuances of the original text while

This interplay between nothingness and creativity is also central to psychoanalytic thought, particularly in the works of Lacan and Žižek. For both, the subject is shaped by its lack, by the void at its core. This lack is not a flaw to be remedied but a structural necessity that generates desire and drives the subject forward. Without this gap, there would be no motivation to seek, to create, or to engage with the world. As Lacan states, "desire is the desire of the Other"—a longing for what lies beyond, for what seems to complete or fulfill us, even though such completion is ultimately unattainable.

This unattainability is not merely a source of frustration; it is the engine of human culture and creativity. The symbolic order, constituted by language, allows us to articulate this desire, giving it form and direction. Yet, as Lacan emphasizes, the symbolic is never sufficient to fully bridge the gap. Language itself is marked by a fundamental impossibility: the inability of signifiers (words) to perfectly correspond to the signified (things or concepts). This slippage between word and thing ensures that desire always persists, opening up space for new interpretations, meanings, and creative acts.

In Bergson's framework, this creative force might be seen as an expression of the *élan vital*—the vital impulse that propels life forward. While Bergson's work does not align perfectly with Lacan's, both thinkers recognize the dynamic interplay between lack and creativity. For Bergson, the drive to create is humanity's response to the intolerability of nothingness. For Lacan, the symbolic order is humanity's means of navigating and negotiating the void.

The Role of Symbolization

Symbolization is central to this process. By transforming the world into a network of signs, language allows us to make sense of our experiences and construct a sense of self. However, this process is never complete. The gap between signifier and signified, and between word and thing, mirrors the gap within the subject itself. This deficiency—the *manque à être*—is not merely a negative condition but a productive one, enabling the symbolic order to function and sustain human culture.

At the same time, symbolization protects us from the overwhelming nature of the Real. In Lacanian terms, the Real is that which resists symbolization, the unassimilable core of existence that threatens to destabilize our constructed realities. Like Perseus using a shield to avoid Medusa's gaze, we use language to mediate our encounter with the Real. This mediation allows us to engage with the world without being overwhelmed by its raw, unfiltered intensity.

The symbolic order also provides a means of confronting and managing the fear of death—the ultimate manifestation of nothingness. Through rituals, narratives, and cultural practices, humans have developed ways of symbolizing mortality, transforming it into something that can be articulated and, to some extent, integrated into life. This does not eliminate the fear of death but channels it into forms that are more bearable and often more meaningful.

Dialectics of Nothingness and Being

Returning to Bergson's question—*Why is there something rather than nothing?*—we see that the relationship between nothingness and being is not one of opposition but of interdependence. Nothingness is not merely the absence of being but an active force that shapes and defines it. Without nothingness, there would be no space for creativity, no impetus for desire, and no motivation to engage with the world.

This dialectical relationship is evident in both Bergson's and Lacan's work. For Bergson, the *élan vital* is humanity's response to the void, a creative force that transforms absence into presence. For Lacan, the symbolic order is humanity's means of navigating the gap, a system that allows us to live with—and even thrive within—the constraints of our lack.

Žižek extends this dialectic into the realm of ideology and culture. He argues that the illusions we construct—whether through religion, art, or politics—are not merely falsehoods to be unmasked but necessary fictions that enable us to function. These illusions provide a framework for making sense of the world, even as they remain incomplete and contingent. The challenge, according to Žižek, is not to eliminate these illusions but to engage with them critically, recognizing both their necessity and their limitations.

Žižek and the Transcendental

Žižek defends a transcendental dialectical materialism of the subject, drawing on the work of Kant and Hegel. The central question concerns the precedence of matter or void. As an idealist within the framework of dialectical materialism, Žižek asserts that the void precedes matter (Žižek, 2012). In contrast, Pippin prefers matter as the initial point of origin (Pippin, 2018). Alternatively, one might argue that both the void and matter co-exist simultaneously, affirming the very essence of dialectics itself (Johnston, 2014).

In the Anglo-Saxon philosophical tradition, the predominant view is that of a materialist starting point, from which evolution leads to complexity, including consciousness. This raises the question: does the mind emerge naturally from nature? From a transcendental perspective, this notion invites skepticism, as it seems to bypass the epistemological and ontological problematics involved in explaining how the transcendental arises from the empirical.

Personally, I lean toward an idealist position, but the genesis of the transcendental remains a profound enigma for me.

Žižek on Contingency and Necessity

Žižek eloquently captures the dialectical interplay between contingency and necessity:

> Any necessity (whether formal, real, or absolute) is a subsequent result arising from or supervening on a prior contingency—specifically, a merely possible actuality just so happening to also enjoy being-there/existence.
>
> *(Žižek, 2012, p. 108)*

> Hegel is … the ultimate thinker of autopoiesis, of the process of the emergence of necessary features out of chaotic contingency, the thinker of contingency's gradual self-organization, of the gradual rise of order out of chaos.
>
> *(Žižek, 2012, p. 108)*

These passages illustrate Žižek's Hegelian appropriation of contingency as the groundless ground of necessity, where the dialectical unfolding reveals the self-organizing power of contradiction.

The Transcendental and the Material

How is it possible for something transcendental to emerge from matter? This fundamental question challenges both idealist and materialist paradigms. If such a genesis were objectively demonstrable, it would imply the potential to create in the laboratory something that is simultaneously material and mental—a synthesis of body and mind.

When this body–mind problematic is transposed to linguistics, the tension persists between the first-person perspective and the third-person perspective inherent in materialism. Johnston critiques this as a false dilemma, arguing that such a shift merely displaces the problem onto another domain of thought:

> The gap between the "social," à la historical materialism, and the "material," à la dialectical materialism, is not to be closed.
>
> *(Johnston, 2014)*

Johnston's analysis foregrounds the irreducibility of dialectical tensions, whether they manifest in epistemology, metaphysics, or socio-historical contexts. This tension, central to Hegelian and post-Hegelian thought, resists any simplistic reduction or synthesis, underscoring the dynamic nature of dialectical processes.

Dialectics and the Transcendental Subject

In light of the above, one might turn to Kant's concept of apperception to interrogate the transcendental status of the subject. For Kant, the "I think" must accompany all representations, establishing a unity of self-consciousness. Žižek, however, radicalizes this notion, emphasizing the void at the heart of subjectivity—the subject as a lack, a non-coincidence with itself. This void aligns with Hegel's concept of the negativity that drives dialectical development.

Similarly, Hegel's notion of the subject as a self-relating negativity finds resonance in Žižek's articulation of the transcendental as rooted in the dialectical interplay between absence and presence, chaos and order. Pippin's insistence on the primacy of material conditions adds a critical counterpoint, suggesting that transcendence cannot be disentangled from immanence.

Conclusion

The unresolved tension between materialism and idealism, body and mind, and first-person and third-person perspectives remains a fertile ground for philosophical inquiry. While Žižek and Johnston champion the dialectical as irreducible and non-reconcilable, the question of the transcendental's genesis within the material continues to challenge and inspire thought.

Creativity and the Future

The creative response to nothingness is not limited to individual acts of art or thought; it also shapes the trajectory of human history. From the development of language to the construction of civilizations, humanity's greatest achievements can be seen as attempts to grapple with the void. Yet these achievements are always provisional, subject to revision and reinterpretation as new challenges arise.

This dynamic process is both a source of hope and a reminder of our limitations. While the symbolic order allows us to construct meaning and navigate the world, it can never fully resolve the tensions at the heart of existence. The gap between being and nothingness remains, ensuring that human life is always in flux, always open to new possibilities.

Bergson's emphasis on creativity and Lacan's focus on desire converge in their recognition of this openness. Both thinkers challenge us to embrace the uncertainty and incompleteness of life, seeing it not as a deficit but as a condition of possibility. By engaging with the void—through art, philosophy, relationships, and action—we can transform absence into presence, creating lives that are meaningful even in the face of nothingness.

18

GENEALOGY OF CREATION

The separation and alienation inherent in human existence generate a gap that is both unbearable and insurmountable. This void fuels the creative process, compelling individuals to construct meaning despite the inherent impossibility of complete resolution. The myth of Sisyphus serves as an apt metaphor for this cycle of desire and creativity, reflecting the ongoing tension that sustains human life.

What does the creative process of the artist have in common with the genesis of the subject when creating something? The confrontation with nothingness. The painter stands before a blank canvas, and the sculptor faces a rough block of marble. The artist cannot tolerate this emptiness and is sometimes even paralyzed by it, as we know from writer's block.

The phenomenon of destruction likely stems from the artist's dissatisfaction with the achieved result: it has fallen far short of the goal he or she had envisioned. Here, parallels with the subject's psychic development begin to emerge. The identity that is achieved leads to dissatisfaction and a longing for something else, which in turn leads to yet another disappointment.

Reverting to nothingness can be understood as the failure of language, which should serve as a shield against the confrontation with the Real.

How often are we confronted with the phenomenon of artists, particularly visual artists, destroying their own work? They aim to express something that cannot be put into words. It seems too simplistic to assume that they destroy their artwork solely because they are dissatisfied with the result. There must be a deeper reason for why this happens. My impression is that it relates to the creative process itself. The unworked block of

DOI: 10.4324/9781003675389-24

marble or the blank canvas exerts an enormous pull, compelling the artist to create something. The emptiness demands to be filled—but with what? A line, an image, a figure? What makes a shape so intriguing? What is it about the filled void that is so alluring? Is it the meaning it conveys? Does the artwork carry symbolic value?

In figurative art, the work of art still refers to something—a figure, an event, a story, or something else. But in non-figurative, abstract art, the element of meaning seems less apparent. Often, the artist themselves cannot articulate the meaning of their work, even though it may resonate deeply with spectators, sometimes due to their knowledge of the artist's tumultuous life, as revealed in interviews. What void is being filled here? Whose void is it—that of the artist or the spectator? How do transference and countertransference play into this dynamic? These are complex questions without easy answers.

According to Lacan, perception and emotion belong to the domain of the Imaginary, while everything that carries meaning resides in the domain of language—the Symbolic (Lacan, 1966). Lacan also claims that the Symbolic achieves the highest form of sublimation, as seen in poetry. A characteristic of the Symbolic is that it exists further from the Real than perception within the Imaginary. This creates a paradox: the greater the distance from the Real, as with the Symbolic, the more urgent creativity becomes. One might expect the opposite. This paradox is especially evident in religions, where the names and stories of gods hold greater significance than their images. Sacred texts such as the Bible, the Quran, and the Torah exemplify this. In the Jewish tradition, there is even a prohibition against speaking God's name aloud, leaving that space open as the ultimate emptiness.

Since humanity first acquired language, there has been an irrepressible urge to name everything: living beings, nature, events, and even things that cannot be perceived. This drive to symbolize knows no bounds. It often runs rampant, as seen in the fanaticism with which cultural and religious groups have fought each other throughout history. More recently, ideologies like fascism and communism have played a significant role in similar conflicts.

An individual's identity is derived from the Other, making them fundamentally a member of the group to which they belong. Identity comes from outside, not from within. The void in the individual is filled externally. Identity is primarily a symbolic construct, colored by the Imaginary of perception. When groups with different cultural or religious backgrounds meet, the differences between them are starkly noticeable because they touch on the core of each group member's identity. When these groups confront one another, violent and aggressive outbursts often follow. The inability to tolerate differences manifests in conversion rage, holy wars, and genocide. Both sides continually refer to the "truth," which each claims to possess.

History, across all continents and cultures, reveals this pattern, continuing into the present day (Achterhuis, 2021). Consider the fanaticism of IS terrorism or the U.S. military interventions in the Middle East.

In reflecting on these ideas, I am inevitably influenced by my Roman Catholic background, in which religious tradition played a significant role. Biblical stories were part of this tradition but were less central than in Protestant traditions. Throughout my academic career, I frequently engaged with individuals from other denominations, learning to appreciate their perspectives while also setting boundaries for myself. The Bible often felt incomprehensible to me, with its agonizing paradoxes and truths that seemed to demand skepticism. Yet, when I read in the Gospel of John, "In the beginning was the Word," I cannot help but think that before that, there was nothing—a great void. Did everything begin with the Word that sought to fill that void, marking the start of something? Did the Word make everything possible—its fancies, developments, the existence of something rather than nothing, and later the dichotomies of good and evil, presence and absence, and the present and the past?

How often are we confronted with the phenomenon of artists—particularly visual artists—destroying their own work? They aim to express something that cannot be captured in words. It seems overly simplistic to assume they destroy their artwork merely because they are dissatisfied with the result. There must be a deeper reason for this behavior. My impression is that it relates to the creative process itself. The unworked block of marble or the blank canvas exerts an irresistible pull, compelling the artist to create. The emptiness demands to be filled—but with what? A line, an image, a figure? What makes a shape so compelling? What is it about the filled void that is so intriguing? Is it the meaning it conveys? Does the artwork hold symbolic value?

In figurative art, the work refers to something—a figure, an event, or a story. But in non-figurative, abstract art, the element of meaning appears less explicit. Often, even the artist cannot fully articulate the meaning of their work, though spectators may perceive profound significance, sometimes influenced by their knowledge of the artist's tumultuous life as revealed in interviews. What void is being filled here? Whose void is it—that of the artist or the spectator? What role do transference and countertransference play in this dynamic? These are complex questions without simple answers.

According to Lacan, perception and emotion belong to the domain of the Imaginary, while meaning resides in the domain of language—the Symbolic (Lacan, 1966). Lacan also claims that the Symbolic achieves its highest form of sublimation in poetry. A characteristic of the Symbolic is that it exists further from the Real than perception within the Imaginary. This creates a paradox: the greater the distance from the Real, as in the

Symbolic, the more urgent creativity becomes. One might expect the opposite. This paradox is especially evident in religion, where the names and stories of gods hold greater significance than their images. Sacred texts such as the Bible, the Quran, and the Torah exemplify this. In Jewish tradition, there is even a prohibition against speaking God's name aloud, leaving that space open as the ultimate emptiness.

Since humanity first acquired language, we have felt an irrepressible urge to name everything: living beings, nature, events, and even things that cannot be perceived. This drive to symbolize knows no bounds. It often runs wild, as seen in the fanaticism with which cultural and religious groups have fought one another throughout history. In more recent times, ideologies like fascism and communism have played similar roles in fostering conflict.

An individual's identity is derived from the Other, making them fundamentally a member of the group to which they belong. Identity comes from outside, not from within. The void in the individual is filled externally. Identity is primarily a symbolic construct, shaped by the Imaginary of perception. When groups with different cultural or religious backgrounds meet, their differences are often starkly highlighted because they touch the core of each group member's identity. These encounters frequently lead to violent and aggressive outbursts. The inability to tolerate difference manifests as conversion rage, holy wars, and genocide. Both sides continually refer to "truth," which each claims to possess.

History across all continents and cultures reveals this pattern, persisting into the present day (Achterhuis, 2021). Consider the fanaticism of IS terrorism or the U.S. military interventions in the Middle East.

Reflecting on these ideas, I am inevitably influenced by my Roman Catholic background, where religious tradition played a significant role. Biblical stories were part of this tradition but were less central than in Protestant traditions. Throughout my academic career, I frequently engaged with individuals from other denominations, learning to appreciate their perspectives while also setting boundaries for myself. The Bible often felt incomprehensible to me, filled with agonizing paradoxes and truths that seemed to require a skeptical approach. Yet, when I read in the Gospel of John, "In the beginning was the Word," I cannot help but think that before the Word, there was nothing—a great void. Did everything begin with the Word, a force that sought to fill that void and marked the start of something? Did the Word make everything possible—its developments, dichotomies, and trajectories, such as something versus nothing, good versus evil, and presence following absence?

If John was correct, could God also be an outgrowth of the Word, with time playing a central role? Or did God emerge from nowhere as a *creatio ex nihilo*—creation from nothing?

19

TOWARD A STRUCTURALIST PSYCHIATRY

The mind–body problem remains an eternal challenge, defying simplistic reductionist solutions. Structuralism offers a counterbalance to modern monism by emphasizing the subjective aspects of human experience. By recognizing the limits and impossibilities inherent in life, structuralism curtails the overconfidence of contemporary scientific approaches that risk excluding the subject altogether. Psychiatry, as a discipline, must make room for the subject if it is to retain its credibility and relevance.

It appears that psychiatry, at the beginning of the 21st century, is increasingly moving toward monistic materialism, driven by the obligation to be scientific. This shift comes at the expense of the subjective aspect.

The structuralist model offers a broader perspective, incorporating not only the somatic but also the psyche, which in its development mirrors and identifies with the structure of its environment. This approach can encompass far more than current psychiatry allows. To avoid the bankruptcy of psychiatry, a broader view—such as the one advocated by structuralism—can be of great value in understanding the psychiatric patient.

In psychiatric practice, an open dialogue is essential, both among practitioners and their teams, as well as in their interactions with patients and the systems of which they are a part. Speaking and listening reflect the desire by which people live. Without desire, life becomes a dead affair.

Over the centuries, psychiatry has primarily focused on the medical model. This focus, in itself, does not necessarily pose serious problems, but when the model is applied too rigidly and one-sidedly, it turns against itself and suffocates in its own praxis. This tendency seems to be becoming evident at the beginning of the 21st century.

DOI: 10.4324/9781003675389-25

Like many human-centered disciplines, psychiatry undergoes cyclical shifts in focus, with emphasis placed on one aspect or another over time. This is influenced by social dynamics and by the fact that humans are complex beings who cannot simply be reduced to a single dimension. The most fundamental and commonly discussed division is that of body and mind, and psyche and soma. Other classifications are also possible: by sex—man or woman; by age—infant, child, adolescent, adult, or elderly; by profession—worker, scholar, soldier, or fisherman; or by social function—politician, judge, manager, and so on. Among these, the most elemental division seems to be that of the psychological and the physical, aspects that are relevant for every individual regardless of their role in society. This fundamental division also forms the essential orientation of psychiatry. Psychiatry views the patient as a human being with a body, behavior, and subjective experiences. These categories cannot simply be reduced to one of these three dimensions. Behavior and experiences reveal psychological aspects that cannot be ignored.

When a psychiatrist regards the body as the sole object of examination and treatment, they make a serious mistake with potentially disastrous consequences.

In this book, I aim to demonstrate that humans are beings who not only possess a body and psyche but also live within a context that structures them and provides them with identity and consciousness. This observation—that identity and consciousness are shaped by context—is not widely accepted in our time. Many believe that these qualities arise spontaneously from the body, particularly the brain. This belief projects all human faculties onto the brain, a view that is too simplistic to be accurate. Yet this reductive representation is gaining popularity in medical circles. Even within psychoanalysis, there are those who attempt to locate consciousness—and even the unconscious—in specific parts of the brain. It should be clear that I do not share this view, and throughout this book, I have highlighted my concerns to the reader.

In my exploration of the essence of humanity, I encountered a black hole, a void. The Real of the body reveals a profound lacuna. However, this does not mean that humans themselves are nothing. On the contrary, humanity's condition is defined by possessing a body that carries a fundamental lack, a void that demands to be filled. Yet this "filling" is not material in nature.

Structuralists have developed a model for understanding this, rooted in the symbolic order—a framework that transcends materiality and is unmistakably embedded in a social context.

In the preceding chapters, I have attempted to outline this structuralist model, guided by thinkers such as René Descartes, Ferdinand de Saussure,

Martin Heidegger, Jacques Lacan, Michel Foucault, and Slavoj Žižek. Each of these thinkers has contributed, in their own way, to this new mode of thought, which has gained traction in sociological and philosophical circles but remains largely absent from medical discourse. This is unfortunate, as the structuralist model is far better equipped to address the complexity of human existence—particularly in the case of individuals with psychological issues. This model could also help psychiatry overcome its current impasse, evident in the widespread dissatisfaction with healthcare in general and psychiatry in particular. This discontent increasingly extends to mental health care professionals themselves. Modern psychiatry lacks an adequate response to the *Uncanny* in Western society, largely due to its one-sided orientation.

The structuralist model discussed here will likely find little resonance in our materialistic civilization. We remain excessively focused on realizing our fantasies and desires, tolerating no limitations in the process. This model may be unpopular because it asserts that humans are not masters of their own bodies, that desire is inherently limited, and that the subject experiences a void that can only be filled with something immaterial. In short, the structuralist model reveals humanity as fundamentally flawed—a "sick animal" that must contend with its lack and survive in the face of nothingness.

Despite this seemingly bleak premise, I do not wish to conclude this book with a purely pessimistic view. On the contrary, it is precisely this lack within human beings that opens up possibilities for joy and extraordinary creativity. The act of filling the void—of addressing this emptiness—offers the opportunity to unlock unprecedented potential and possibilities.

This version improves clarity, coherence, and flow while preserving the depth and nuance of

The structuralist perspective illuminates the human condition in a way that transcends the narrow confines of the medical model. It views the human subject as inherently shaped by language, culture, and social structures—elements that do not fit neatly into a purely biological or materialist framework. This model suggests that human identity and consciousness are not merely the result of brain activity but are deeply rooted in the symbolic systems that structure our lives. These systems shape how we perceive ourselves, relate to others, and understand the world.

The Role of the Symbolic in Psychiatry

By emphasizing the symbolic order, the structuralist model provides a richer understanding of psychological issues. Many psychiatric disorders, such as anxiety, depression, and psychosis, cannot be fully explained by biological dysfunction alone. These conditions often reflect disturbances in the subject's relationship with the symbolic order, manifesting as feelings of alienation, fragmentation, or lack of meaning. For example, Lacan's concept of the *manque à être* (*lack of being*) highlights how the subject is fundamentally defined by a sense of incompleteness—a void that drives desire but can also lead to suffering when misaligned with the symbolic structures that give life coherence.

In this sense, structuralism offers psychiatry a way to move beyond symptom management toward a deeper engagement with the existential and symbolic dimensions of human experience. This approach is not about rejecting biology or the medical model but about integrating these with a broader understanding of what it means to be human. Such integration could address the growing dissatisfaction with psychiatry's inability to grapple with the deeper, non-material aspects of mental health.

The Crisis in Modern Psychiatry

The dissatisfaction with contemporary psychiatry is not limited to patients but extends to practitioners themselves. Mental health professionals increasingly report feelings of burnout and frustration, often tied to the constraints of a system that prioritizes efficiency, diagnosis, and pharmacological treatment over meaningful engagement with patients. The structuralist model, with its emphasis on the symbolic and the social, could offer a way out of this crisis by reintroducing a more humanistic and holistic perspective into psychiatric practice.

At its core, the structuralist approach challenges the idea that human suffering can be fully understood or alleviated through material means alone. It argues that the void at the center of human existence—the *manque à être*—cannot be filled with medication, therapy, or material achievements. Instead, this lack must be navigated through symbolic engagement, creativity, and connection with others. By recognizing this, psychiatry could reclaim its role as a discipline that addresses not just the biological but also the existential and symbolic dimensions of mental health.

Humanity's Relationship with the Void

The void, far from being a purely negative force, is what makes human creativity and desire possible. It is the gap between what we are and what we aspire to be, between what we have and what we long for, that drives innovation, art, and personal growth. Structuralist thinkers like Lacan and Žižek argue that this void is not a flaw but a defining feature of the human condition. Without it, there would be no desire, no movement, and no creation.

This perspective transforms the void from something to be feared or eradicated into something to be embraced and explored. The void is not a sign of failure or inadequacy but a space of potential. It is the foundation of human creativity, as seen in art, literature, and even scientific discovery. By filling the void with symbolic meaning, humans find ways to make life bearable, meaningful, and even joyful.

Toward a New Psychiatry

Integrating structuralist insights into psychiatry would require a shift in focus from solely addressing symptoms to exploring the deeper symbolic and existential dimensions of mental health. This does not mean abandoning the medical model but rather complementing it with a broader framework that recognizes the complexity of the human condition. Such an approach would involve the following:

1. **Acknowledging the Role of the Symbolic:** Understanding how language, culture, and social structures shape identity and mental health.
2. **Addressing the Void:** Recognizing the *manque à être* as a central feature of human existence and helping patients navigate it creatively rather than suppressing or ignoring it.
3. **Promoting Holistic Care:** Balancing biological interventions with therapies that engage the symbolic and relational dimensions of the patient's experience.
4. **Empowering Practitioners:** Providing mental health professionals with tools and frameworks to address the existential and symbolic aspects of their patients' suffering, reducing burnout and increasing job satisfaction.
5. **Resisting Reductionism:** Challenging the dominance of materialist and reductionist perspectives in psychiatry by fostering dialogue between medical, sociological, and philosophical disciplines.

A Hopeful Conclusion

Despite its seemingly bleak premise, the structuralist view of humanity offers a hopeful perspective. It acknowledges human limitations and flaws while highlighting the incredible potential for creativity and transformation that arises from these very deficiencies. The void at the heart of the human condition is not a problem to be solved but a mystery to be engaged with—a source of inspiration, possibility, and growth.

By embracing this perspective, psychiatry could not only address the current crisis in mental health care but also reimagine itself as a discipline that fully acknowledges the depth and complexity of human experience. In doing so, it could offer patients and practitioners alike a more meaningful and fulfilling way to navigate the challenges of modern life.

20

THE ROLE OF LINGUISTICS IN A THERAPEUTIC PERSPECTIVE

Structuralism places language at the core of human reality, presenting it as a network that shapes how we perceive and interact with the world. This system of rules and structures is inseparable from human experience. It draws a clear distinction between physical reality and the symbolic system of language, underscoring its centrality in shaping human perception. Particularly in psychiatry, and especially in cases of psychosis, disruptions in this semiotic system highlight the fragility of linguistic order. Therapy must address these disruptions by engaging with the dialectical relationship between speaking and listening. Speaking sustains desire, making the therapist's role as an attentive listener indispensable in the therapeutic process.

Structuralism, pioneered by Ferdinand de Saussure, revolutionized the understanding of language and influenced numerous disciplines within the humanities, including anthropology, psychoanalysis, and philosophy. While structuralism developed predominantly in Western Europe, particularly in France, Russian formalism emerged concurrently in the Soviet Union. Figures such as Julia Kristeva and Tzvetan Todorov bridged these intellectual traditions, and the Russian linguistic tradition found a unique voice in Mikhail Bakhtin.

Bakhtin opposed the rigid formalism of his contemporaries, critiquing structuralism for overly mechanistic interpretations of language. His later work, *Towards a Philosophy of the Act*, reflects influences from the neo-Kantian Marburg school, represented by Hermann Cohen and Ernst Cassirer (Bakhtin, 1993). By the 1980s, Bakhtin's focus on the social and practical aspects of language gained recognition in France, the United States, and the United Kingdom. His concept of "outsideness," also called

DOI: 10.4324/9781003675389-26

"extopy" in Western contexts, captures the relational dynamics of language. This idea resonates with Lacan's psychoanalytic theory, despite the two thinkers never having met.

A personal encounter with Jaakko Seikkula deepened my interest in Bakhtin's work, particularly its connections to French structuralism and Russian formalism. This inspired a reevaluation of Bakhtin's ideas in the context of the crisis of the subject. As Mariya Kalinova succinctly puts it:

> Mikhail Bakhtin and Jacques Lacan, though belonging to distinct intellectual traditions, share a critical stance against dominant discourses—Soviet totalitarianism in Bakhtin's case, and Western capitalism in Lacan's. Both critique the constitution of truth as an absolute category and emphasize the subject's capacity to construct autonomous meaning.
>
> *(Kalinova, 2018)*

Central to both Bakhtin and Lacan are the concepts of "outsideness" and "extimacy." For Bakhtin, outsideness refers to the idea that the subject is always partially understood through the perspective of the Other. Similarly, Lacan's concept of extimacy highlights how the subject's sense of self is shaped by external forces—particularly the discourse of the Other. Both thinkers converge on the notion that self-understanding arises through interaction, whether in dialogue (Bakhtin) or through the symbolic order of language (Lacan).

This dynamic is evident in Sartre's *L'Imaginaire* (1940), where he describes perception as incomplete—seeing only parts of a cube while the rest must be imagined. Similarly, in understanding oneself, the subject encounters a lack that can only be addressed through the Other. Lacan capitalized this "Other" to emphasize its role as a mirror reflecting the subject's incompleteness, a dynamic that operates not only in perception but also in the deeper processes of self-experience.

For therapy, this means that identity and self-experience are inherently relational. The presence of the Other, often represented by the therapist, is crucial for the help-seeker to articulate their identity. Listening, in this context, is not a passive act but an active engagement that allows the patient's narrative to emerge.

Lacan's notion of extimacy, first defined in his 1960 seminar, reflects this dynamic: "What we described as the central place, as the intimate exteriority or extimacy, that is the Thing." (Lacan, 1992, p. 139).

Therapeutic listening, however, is often hindered by caregivers prioritizing their expertise over the patient's voice. Biological interventions, while sometimes helpful, can suppress this dialogical process rather than foster it. Dialogue becomes essential in helping the subject to emerge, as speaking is the very act that constitutes the self.

Bakhtin's interpretation of Freud's unconscious further illustrates this point. For Bakhtin, the unconscious is external and shaped through interaction with the outside world. This contrasts with Freud's view of the unconscious as deeply internal and hidden. Bakhtin's focus on dialogue connects seamlessly with Jaakko Seikkula's open dialogue method, where the caregiver refrains from assuming the role of an all-knowing authority and instead listens with curiosity and respect for the patient's narrative (Seikkula, 2022).

Jakobson, Bakhtin, and Lacan: A Convergence

Roman Jakobson's linguistic theories bridge Russian formalism and French structuralism, influencing figures like Lévi-Strauss and Lacan. His concept of "markedness" and focus on the relational aspects of language align with both Bakhtin's dialogism and Lacan's symbolic order. Jakobson's emphasis on the interplay between signifiers informed Lacan's assertion that "the unconscious is structured like a language."

Both Jakobson and Bakhtin view language as inherently interactive. For Bakhtin, meaning emerges through dialogue between speaker and listener, a process Jakobson highlights in the relational functions of language. This aligns with Lacan's concept of the Other, which shapes the subject's identity through discourse.

The Crisis of the Subject

All three thinkers challenge the Enlightenment ideal of the autonomous subject. For Bakhtin, outsideness reveals the subject's dependence on the Other for self-understanding. Lacan's extimacy underscores this relationality, emphasizing that the subject is shaped by gaps and absences in the symbolic order. Jakobson complements this critique by showing how meaning arises from relational differences within language, rather than from any inherent essence.

Implications for Therapy

These insights underscore the importance of dialogue in therapy. The help-seeker's self-discovery depends on the caregiver's active listening and willingness to engage without imposing authority. Lacan's extimacy and Bakhtin's dialogism converge in the open dialogue method, which prioritizes the patient's voice and narrative over predefined solutions.

Outside and Inside: A Dialectical Bridge

Ultimately, Bakhtin, Jakobson, and Lacan dismantle the rigid boundary between inside and outside. Identity, they argue, is a dynamic process shaped by relational forces. This dialectic between self and Other and between inside and outside becomes a bridge that enables the subject to articulate their place in the world and to engage with it meaningfully.

21

THE ECLIPSE OF THE (PSYCHOTIC) SUBJECT?

Throughout this book, I have highlighted the risks of science's exclusive focus on objectivity, which often leads to the erasure of the subject. Will the subject eventually disappear entirely from our understanding of reality? Foucault entertains this possibility, envisioning a future devoid of subjectivity. Personally, I find such a vision unsettling. Without the subject, there can be no thought or reflection. The psychotic subject, too, would cease to exist, leaving an empty void where meaning once resided.

Thinking and speaking are conditions of life for the subject. When speaking and listening fade away, the death instinct will gain the upper hand, and the subject will perish. As practitioners and as human beings, we must resist this—not only in relation to our patients but also in relation to ourselves—otherwise, we are doomed to die. In our time, engaging in open dialogue with others must be given the highest priority.

In my search of psychiatric literature for the keyword "self," I found almost no references to the term. I was disappointed. It was no better with the keywords "I" and "subject," though psychoanalytically and phenomenologically oriented publications provided some exceptions. What could this signify? To me, it suggests an overemphasis on the "scientific" orientation within psychiatry and certain branches of psychoanalysis—an overemphasis that downplays the reflective and psychological dimensions of psychiatry.

Where has the concept of the self gone in professional literature? Has there ever been attention to the self, the "I," or the subject in psychiatry? Undoubtedly, but any such interest seems to have largely vanished for now.

DOI: 10.4324/9781003675389-27

To understand the role of the self within and outside psychiatry, we must turn to philosophy. Philosophy abounds with texts dealing with the self and the subject. For instance, Foucault speaks of the disappearance of the subject in Western culture just centuries after Descartes discovered it. Lacan explores the self's place in the symbolic order through his "graphe," while Deleuze and Guattari examine it through the rhizomatic structure of interactional networks.

The place of psychosis within this development will also be addressed here. The following questions arise: Can the psychotic no longer find their place within this labyrinth? Does a self exist within the psychotic experience? Or does the psychotic attempt to obscure their own self? These questions will form the core of this discussion.

The Self in a Structural Perspective

Recently, I reread Michel Foucault's *The Discourse on Language* (*L'ordre du discours*), and for the second time, I was shaken by the implications of his work. My first shock came from the final sentence of his *The Order of Things* (*Les mots et les choses*, 1966). After tracing the development of the human sciences, Foucault writes:

> If these dispositions were to disappear as they appeared, if they were to vanish because of an event we can only imagine the possibility of, but whose form we cannot yet predict—as the ground of classical thought vanished at the end of the 18th century—then one can certainly wager that man would be erased, like a face drawn in the sand at the edge of the sea.
>
> *(Foucault, 1966)*

This chilling assertion points to the possibility of a world without the self, the subject, or humanity. Such a scenario would also lack anyone to document it, as well as the means to document it. Was Foucault offering a prediction or issuing a warning? I find it difficult to imagine such a world, except perhaps in the event of a global nuclear catastrophe. Let us hope such a disaster never comes to pass.

The second shock came from *The Discourse on Language*, which Foucault delivered as an inaugural lecture at the Collège de France on December 2, 1970. Toward the end of the lecture, Foucault outlines the philosopher's task: to dismantle the systems of meaning so that only things and events remain. What was tentative in *The Order of Things*—the suggestion that humanity might disappear from the world stage—becomes more explicit here, even taking the form of a directive: abolish the system of meaning.

This demand strikes at the root of humanity itself. Without meaning systems, language—the most prominent system of meaning—would vanish. With it would go thought, communication, and consciousness. We would become mere things among things, or animals among animals, or at most robots.

A Structuralist Framework for Psychiatry

This introduction to Foucault's discourse serves as a springboard for discussing a structuralist approach to psychiatry, which will include an exploration of the self, the disappearance of the subject, and ways to address it. Some elements may seem familiar, while others may feel alien. Though theoretical, I assure you this framework has strong practical relevance. As the saying goes: "There is nothing more practical than a good theory."

The Linguistic Foundations of Structuralism

De Saussure's most basic unit of language, the linguistic sign—as we have seen—consists of two parts: the *signified* (an idea or concept) and the *signifier* (the spoken or written word). These two elements are interconnected but do not possess inherent meaning in isolation. Instead, meaning emerges through the relationship between signs.

In the structuralist view, the self is one such object. Through language, the subject can refer to themselves, presenting both their physical body and intangible qualities such as a name, personality, or role. Thus, the self has two dimensions: the tangible body and its symbolic representation. This symbolic aspect allows for self-awareness and the emergence of identity. Language acts as a mirror, enabling the subject to recognize and construct their self.

Without language, the self would not exist. Language predates the individual; it is a structure into which the child is born. As Lacan puts it, the "Other"—representing the symbolic order—exists before the subject. Gradually, through interaction with caregivers, the child begins to integrate into this symbolic world, adopting the language and cultural frameworks of their environment.

The Self and Psychosis

What happens to the self in psychosis? Drawing on Lacan's concept of "foreclosure," we see that psychosis often involves a rejection of the symbolic order. This rejection disrupts the integration of language, identity, and self-awareness. Without the mediating function of the symbolic, the psychotic is left adrift in the Imaginary, unable to distinguish fully between fantasy and reality.

The psychotic's relationship with the Other is also fractured. Take Louis Wolfson, who rejected his native English by inventing a method of instantly translating spoken English into other languages to shield himself from its perceived intrusion (Wolfson, 1970). His case illustrates the desperate measures psychotics may take to construct autonomy by excluding the Other. Yet such defenses often leave the subject isolated and alienated.

Through this exploration of the self, it becomes clear that the self is deeply intertwined with language, the symbolic order, and the Other. The self is not an independent entity but an emergent phenomenon—a reflection shaped by time and interaction.

Modern psychiatry, however, risks erasing the subject by fixating on objectivity and biological reductionism. While biological psychiatry has its place, it must remain balanced with an understanding of the structural and symbolic dimensions of human existence. Psychiatry must retain a space for the subject, lest it devolve into a purely neurological practice.

Patients like Louis Wolfson remind us of the necessity of maintaining dialogue, both with our patients and with the broader symbolic structures that constitute humanity. Only by staying in dialogue can we prevent the disappearance of the subject.

The Subject in Modern Psychiatry

In modern psychiatry, the concept of the subject—the self—is increasingly sidelined in favor of measurable, observable phenomena. Biological psychiatry, which focuses on brain chemistry, neural networks, and genetics, dominates the field. While these approaches yield valuable insights, their singular focus risks reducing the human experience to mere biological functions. Psychiatry, if it is to remain relevant and holistic, must acknowledge the complexity of human existence. It must integrate the biological with the symbolic, the subjective, and the cultural.

The structuralist approach, as outlined here, provides a way to restore the subject to psychiatry. By recognizing the fundamental role of language, the symbolic order, and the Other in shaping identity and self-awareness, psychiatry can address the deeper dimensions of mental health. Structuralism reminds us that the self is not a static entity but a dynamic process that unfolds in dialogue with others and the world.

The Crisis of the Self in Psychosis

Psychosis exemplifies the crisis of the self when the symbolic order collapses. In psychosis, the subject loses its anchor in language and struggles to differentiate between reality and fantasy. This collapse is not merely a breakdown of brain function but a profound disruption in the symbolic structures that enable self-awareness and coherence.

Lacan's concept of "foreclosure" (*forclusion*) provides a useful lens to understand psychosis. Foreclosure refers to the rejection of the Name-of-the-Father, the symbolic law that mediates the transition from the Imaginary to the Symbolic order. Without this mediation, the psychotic is unable to fully integrate into the shared symbolic framework, leaving them isolated and vulnerable to the overwhelming forces of the Real.

The case of Louis Wolfson illustrates this dynamic. His rejection of his mother tongue and creation of an alternative linguistic system can be seen as an attempt to construct autonomy in the absence of a stable symbolic foundation. While this strategy offered temporary relief, it ultimately left him alienated and disconnected.

Toward a Structuralist Psychiatry

Structuralist psychiatry offers a path forward by emphasizing the importance of the symbolic order in mental health. Rather than viewing psychosis purely as a biological disorder, this approach recognizes it as a disruption in the subject's relationship with the symbolic, the Imaginary, and the Other. By addressing these dimensions, psychiatry can provide more meaningful and effective interventions.

A structuralist approach would entail the following:

1. **Reintegrating the Subject:** Psychiatry must make space for the subject by acknowledging the role of language, culture, and relationships in shaping identity and self-awareness.
2. **Balancing the Biological and Symbolic:** While biological treatments have their place, they must be complemented by therapies that engage the symbolic and relational dimensions of the patient's experience.
3. **Fostering Dialogue:** Psychiatric practice should prioritize dialogue, both with patients and within the field itself. This means listening to patients as subjects, not merely treating them as objects of observation.
4. **Resisting Reductionism:** Psychiatry must resist the temptation to reduce human experience to neural processes alone. Instead, it should embrace the complexity and richness of the human condition.

Preserving the Subject in Psychiatry

The disappearance of the subject from psychiatry reflects a broader cultural trend toward objectification and quantification. In this context, structuralist psychiatry offers a counterbalance. It reminds us that the self is not a thing to be measured but a dynamic process that unfolds through language, relationships, and reflection.

If psychiatry is to remain a humanistic discipline, it must defend the subject against the encroachments of reductionism. This means engaging with the complex interplay of biology, culture, and language that shapes human existence. It also means staying in dialogue—with patients, with colleagues, and with the broader cultural and intellectual currents that inform our understanding of the self.

Patients like Louis Wolfson remind us of the stakes of this work. They show us the fragility of the self and the profound importance of the symbolic order in sustaining it. By listening to their stories and engaging with their struggles, we can learn to navigate the challenges of modern psychiatry while preserving its core mission: to care for the whole person, not just their symptoms.

As Foucault warned, the disappearance of the subject would mark the end of humanity as we know it. To prevent this, we must resist the forces that seek to erase the self—from reductionist science to cultural and political pressures that devalue individuality. By embracing a structuralist perspective, psychiatry can reclaim its role as a discipline that values the complexity and depth of human experience.

Let us stay in dialogue. Let us listen to our patients and to one another. In doing so, we can ensure that the subject—and the self—remains at the heart of psychiatry.

The Role of Desire and Speaking in the Self

Lacan famously declared that "the unconscious is structured like a language." In this statement, the intricate relationship between desire, speaking, and the self becomes apparent. Desire, for Lacan, is not merely a longing for material or emotional satisfaction but a force rooted in the very structure of language and the symbolic order. It emerges from a fundamental lack—a void created by the separation from the Real and our entry into the Symbolic.

Desire: The Product of Lack

Lacan's notion of desire begins with the *manque à être*—the "lack of being." This lack is inherent to the human condition and is introduced by the symbolic order when the subject separates from the Real (the prelinguistic state). Desire is not directed toward fulfilling this lack in a definitive way; instead, it perpetuates itself through symbolic substitutions, driven by an endless pursuit of meaning and connection.

When a child enters language, they step into the domain of the Other, adopting the signifiers that constitute identity and communication. Yet this entry into language comes at a cost: the loss of the Real and the impossibility of full self-presence. The subject is barred (*le sujet barré*), existing as a fragmented self within the web of language and culture. This fragmentation creates a gap between the subject and its own being—a gap that gives rise to desire.

Speaking as the Articulation of Desire

If desire is born from the lack introduced by the Symbolic, then speaking becomes its primary mode of articulation. Speech allows the subject to give voice to their longing, not as a direct expression of need but as a mediated attempt to fill the void through symbolic means. This makes speaking an act of creation—it brings something into existence by naming it, even if that "something" can never fully satisfy the subject's desire.

Speech, however, is not purely an individual act. It is always addressed to the Other. In fact, desire itself is "the desire of the Other," meaning that the subject's desire is shaped and mediated by their relationship to others within the symbolic order. The Other provides the signifiers through which the subject can articulate their desire, but it also represents the unattainable ideal that the subject continually strives for.

For Lacan, this dynamic is embodied in the *objet petit a*—the unattainable object of desire. The *objet petit a* is not a concrete thing but a placeholder for the lost Real. It drives the subject's pursuit of meaning and connection but can never be fully captured through language or achieved in reality.

Speaking as a Therapeutic Act

In the clinical setting, the act of speaking takes on profound significance. The patient's speech is not merely a recounting of symptoms or experiences; it is an articulation of desire. The role of the therapist, then, is not to provide answers or impose meaning but to listen—to create a space where the patient's desire can unfold.

The therapeutic dialogue becomes a process of co-creation, where the patient and therapist explore the symbolic gaps and misalignments that underlie the patient's suffering. This process is not about achieving closure or resolution but about enabling the subject to engage with their desire in a way that is dynamic and transformative.

For the psychotic, whose relationship with the symbolic order is disrupted, speaking is both an opportunity and a challenge. On the one hand, it allows the psychotic to engage with the Other and attempt to construct meaning. On the other hand, their rejection of the Name-of-the-Father and the resulting foreclosure of key symbolic structures often make this process fraught with difficulty. The therapist's task is to listen without judgment, allowing the psychotic's speech to unfold on its own terms and facilitating the possibility of symbolic reconstruction.

The Link Between Desire, Speaking, and the Self

The self, as explored earlier, is not an inherent or stable entity. It is an emergent phenomenon shaped by the interplay of language, desire, and relationships with others. Desire sustains the self, propelling it forward in its quest for meaning, while speaking provides the medium through which this desire is articulated and explored.

Lacan's concept of *extimacy*—the intimate exteriority of the self—captures this dynamic. The self is not contained within the individual but is constituted in its relationship with the Other. Through speaking, the subject externalizes their inner world, creating a bridge between their fragmented self and the symbolic structures that sustain identity.

This relational and dynamic view of the self challenges the reductionist tendencies of modern psychiatry, which often seeks to localize identity and consciousness within the brain. By ignoring the symbolic and relational dimensions of the self, psychiatry risks overlooking the very mechanisms that make healing and transformation possible.

Desire and Speaking in the Treatment of Psychosis

In psychosis, the breakdown of the symbolic order creates a crisis of desire and speaking. The psychotic subject often becomes trapped in the Imaginary, where fantasy and reality blur, and the symbolic frameworks needed to articulate desire are absent or disrupted. This breakdown can manifest as delusions, hallucinations, or a sense of alienation from the self and others.

Yet even in psychosis, the desire to speak remains. The psychotic's speech may seem fragmented or incoherent to outsiders, but it is nonetheless an attempt to engage with the Other and make sense of their experience. The therapist's role is to meet the psychotic in this fragmented space, listening with openness and curiosity rather than imposing preconceptions or diagnoses.

The therapeutic relationship itself becomes a symbolic bridge, allowing the psychotic subject to re-engage with the symbolic order. Through this process, the psychotic can begin to reconstruct a sense of self and reconnect with their desire in a way that is meaningful and sustainable.

Conclusion: Desire as the Engine of the Self

Desire and speaking are not just aspects of human experience; they are its engine. Without desire, there would be no movement, no growth, and no creativity. Without speaking, there would be no way to give shape to desire, no way to connect with others, and no way to construct a self.

In the face of psychiatry's increasing focus on biology and objectivity, structuralism offers a powerful reminder of the symbolic and relational dimensions of human existence. By embracing these dimensions, psychiatry can preserve its humanistic core and provide care that addresses the full complexity of the subject.

Through dialogue, we can sustain the self. Through listening, we can keep desire alive. And through speaking, we can create a world where the subject not only survives but also thrives.

22

WHAT ABOUT THE SELF?

This book centers on the subjective self, particularly as it relates to psychiatry and psychosis. The subject is under threat, both within psychiatry and beyond. To preserve the (psychotic) subject, we must fundamentally reconsider our understanding of humanity. Psychosis offers an opportunity to confront and restore the subject to our collective consciousness. A structuralist perspective can play a significant role in this process.

The Evolution of the Self: Reflections and Future Perspectives

Throughout this book, we have explored various conceptions of the self. History shows that the self, in the guise of the subject, has had only a brief existence. While manifestations of self-awareness—such as Augustine's *Confessions*—indicate early reflections on the self, it was not until Descartes in the 17th century that explicit reference was made to a self-conscious being, the *res cogitans*.

Since then, numerous philosophers have critiqued or rejected the notion of the subject, including Nietzsche, Husserl, Hegel, Heidegger, Wittgenstein, and Ryle. These rejections often stem from technical-philosophical perspectives tied to the methods employed. Ryle, for example, approached the subject purely through logic, arguing that psychological views of the self are so varied and contradictory that one cannot speak of unity. Husserl moved away from the Cartesian subject-object dualism, and Foucault advocated for an active approach to self-signification. And Wittgenstein? His work further problematized the notion of a unified subject.

DOI: 10.4324/9781003675389-28

To me, these critiques suggest that our understanding of the subject is overdue for serious revision—one that incorporates these criticisms while preserving the essence of the self. It is too simplistic to deny the existence of the self or the subject altogether to accommodate a "pure ontology," as Heidegger envisioned. Such a perspective risks ethical and practical consequences, which are already visible in the world around us.

The Need for a Radical Reevaluation of the Self

It is time to radically rethink our conceptions of the self. A pure ontological approach, while insightful, is insufficient for an adequate understanding of the subject. A solipsistic framing of the self is ethically untenable, as evidenced by contemporary challenges. Consider the rise of individual fantasies shaping reality to personal will—manifesting, for instance, in the ongoing transgender discourse or the broader rejection of limitations and norms. While personal autonomy is critical, unchecked self-centralization risks undermining shared ethical foundations.

The political arena further demonstrates the consequences of solipsistic self-positioning, with figures like Trump and Putin embodying a disregard for collective values. This trend suggests a growing detachment from ethical essences and shared norms.

Additionally, the boundary between "inside" and "outside" the self is no longer as clearly demarcated. As explored throughout this book, the self is as much shaped by the external as by the internal; the two exist in dialectical relationship. Any revised understanding of the subject must account for this interaction.

Transcendence and Structure in the Subject

A crucial dimension of the subject is its capacity for transcendence. Within a structuralist orientation, this transcendent capacity must be understood in terms of its external structuring through language. Language mediates and supports the self, allowing the subject to emerge within the symbolic order. This structuring has been discussed extensively in this book, highlighting the intricate interplay between the symbolic, the Other, and the subject.

Yet the current view of humanity increasingly neglects these nuances, favoring a purely naturalistic perspective. While naturalism offers simplicity, it does a disservice to the complexity of human existence. From a humanistic perspective, such reductionism risks unprecedented political and social catastrophes, as well as profound personal consequences. A life guided solely by the pursuit of pleasure, well-being, and happiness, without a grounding in shared ethical and symbolic frameworks, is unlikely to end well.

Therefore, despite dire predictions and societal temptations, we must hold the subject and the self in high regard. They represent a bulwark against the erosion of meaning and ethical integrity.

The Role of Psychiatry in Preserving the Self

Whether modern psychiatry can accommodate a renewed conception of the self remains an open question. What is clear, however, is that such an accommodation is necessary. Psychiatry must resist the lure of reductive naturalism, which, while straightforward, fails to capture the complexity of the subject.

From my decades of experience working primarily with individuals experiencing psychosis, I have found that engaging with their speech is the most effective way to facilitate improvement. My approach began intuitively, guided by results—small steps and occasional breakthroughs. While I cannot claim to have "cured" patients in a medical-psychiatric sense, I succeeded in establishing meaningful contact with most of them. This process was often slow and met with initial resistance, but persistence yielded connection.

Parents frequently expressed frustration: "You can do it, but we can't." Their reaction is understandable, as the process of building rapport with psychotic patients often requires an extraordinary level of patience and openness.

Speaking, Listening, and the Formation of the Subject

Over time, I complemented my intuitive practice with extensive reading in psychoanalysis, phenomenology, and structuralism. Gradually, it became clear to me that speaking was the most vital instrument for progress—not my speaking, but that of the patient. The act of listening emerged as a fundamental element of this process. Speaking presupposes listening, and listening presupposes the presence of the Other.

With Lacan, I came to understand that "the subject is the effect of speaking." Speaking brings the subject into existence, allowing them to articulate their desires, struggles, and identity. This realization took years to articulate explicitly, but it has become the cornerstone of my practice.

A Path Forward

As we reflect on the trajectory of the self, it is evident that the subject and the self are deeply intertwined with language, the Other, and the symbolic order. The self is not a static entity but a dynamic process, continually shaped and reshaped through dialogue and interaction.

Modern psychiatry must recognize and honor this complexity. A purely naturalistic or reductionist approach cannot account for the richness of the human experience. While biological psychiatry has its place, it must coexist with a structuralist understanding of the subject—one that acknowledges the role of language, desire, and relationality in shaping identity and self-awareness.

In practice, this means prioritizing dialogue with patients, even those who present with severe psychotic symptoms. Speaking and listening remain our most powerful tools for engaging with the subject and facilitating transformation. As practitioners, we must resist the temptation to impose predefined frameworks and instead meet patients where they are, creating space for their voices to emerge.

By preserving the subject and the self within psychiatry, we uphold not only the dignity of our patients but also the integrity of the field itself. Let us remain committed to this dialogue, for it is through speaking and listening that we sustain the subject and nurture the possibilities of human existence.

Objectivism and Subjectivism: Toward a Dialectical Relationship

In contemporary psychiatry and beyond, the opposition between objectivism and subjectivism has reached a critical juncture. Instead of engaging in a productive dialectical relationship, these two perspectives increasingly appear to exclude one another. This polarization poses significant challenges, particularly in the domain of mental health, where both perspectives are essential to understanding and addressing the complexities of human existence.

The Rise of Objectivism

Objectivism, as it manifests in early 21st-century psychiatry, prioritizes measurable phenomena: brain scans, neurotransmitter imbalances, genetic markers, and behavioral data. This approach aligns with the broader trend of scientism, where knowledge is equated with what can be quantified and empirically verified. Psychiatry has embraced objectivism to solidify its status as a medical science, focusing on biological determinants of mental disorders.

The advantages of objectivism are clear. It has led to groundbreaking discoveries in neurobiology, the development of psychotropic medications, and evidence-based practices. These advancements have undoubtedly improved the lives of countless patients. However, the reliance on objectivism has its limitations, particularly when applied uncritically. By reducing human experience to brain chemistry or neural networks, psychiatry risks neglecting the subjective dimensions of suffering—dimensions that cannot be fully captured by empirical data.

The Marginalization of Subjectivism

Subjectivism, which emphasizes the inner experiences, desires, and meanings of the individual, has been increasingly marginalized in psychiatry. While psychoanalysis and phenomenology once held significant sway, their influence has waned in the face of objectivist methodologies. This marginalization is particularly problematic because subjectivism addresses aspects of human existence that objectivism cannot—namely, the lived experience of being.

At its core, subjectivism recognizes that individuals are not merely objects to be studied but subjects who experience, interpret, and shape their worlds. The subjective dimension is where questions of identity, meaning, and desire arise. Neglecting this dimension impoverishes psychiatry, reducing it to a mechanistic practice that fails to address the full complexity of the human condition.

The Need for a Dialectical Relationship

The exclusionary stance between objectivism and subjectivism is not only unproductive but also untenable. These perspectives are not mutually exclusive; rather, they are interdependent and should be understood as part of a dialectical relationship. Objectivism provides the tools to investigate the biological and material underpinnings of mental phenomena, while subjectivism offers insights into the symbolic, relational, and existential dimensions of human experience.

The dialectical relationship between objectivism and subjectivism can be illustrated through the concept of mental health itself. On the one hand, mental health has a biological basis, influenced by genetics, neurochemistry, and physiology. On the other hand, it is profoundly shaped by subjective experiences, cultural contexts, and interpersonal relationships. A holistic understanding of mental health requires both perspectives.

The False Dichotomy in 21st-Century Psychiatry

In the early 21st century, the divide between objectivism and subjectivism has widened, creating a false dichotomy. Objectivism increasingly dominates, often dismissing subjectivism as unscientific or outdated. This exclusionary stance has serious consequences, as it overlooks the richness and complexity of the human experience.

For example, consider the treatment of depression. An objectivist approach might focus exclusively on correcting serotonin imbalances or activating specific neural pathways. While these interventions can be effective, they do not address the subjective dimensions of despair, meaninglessness, or alienation that often accompany depression. A purely objectivist approach risks treating symptoms while ignoring the deeper existential struggles of the patient.

Conversely, a purely subjectivist approach that disregards biological factors is equally flawed. Such an approach might fail to recognize the role of neurochemical imbalances or genetic predispositions in shaping mental health. Without addressing these biological underpinnings, subjective interventions risk being ineffective or incomplete.

A Dialectical Psychiatry: Balancing Objectivism and Subjectivism

To move beyond the current impasse, psychiatry must embrace a dialectical framework that integrates objectivism and subjectivism. This framework acknowledges that human beings are both biological organisms and symbolic beings. It seeks to understand how these dimensions interact and influence one another.

1 **Integration in Diagnosis:** A dialectical approach would consider both biological markers and subjective experiences when diagnosing mental disorders. For instance, while brain imaging can provide valuable insights into structural abnormalities, understanding a patient's personal narrative is equally critical.
2 **Therapeutic Interventions:** Treatment should address both the biological and subjective dimensions of mental health. Medication can alleviate symptoms and stabilize neurochemical imbalances, but therapy must engage with the patient's experiences, desires, and meanings to facilitate deeper healing.
3 **Research Paradigms:** Psychiatric research should adopt methodologies that integrate objectivist and subjectivist perspectives. This might involve combining quantitative studies with qualitative research to capture the full spectrum of human experience.
4 **Ethical Considerations:** A dialectical psychiatry must also address the ethical implications of its practices. Objectivism's focus on standardization and efficiency should not override the subjectivist commitment to individualized care and respect for the patient's autonomy.

Desire and Speaking as a Bridge Between Objectivism and Subjectivism

Desire and speaking offer a conceptual bridge between objectivism and subjectivism. As Lacan famously stated, "The subject is the effect of speaking." This assertion highlights the role of language in shaping identity, meaning, and desire. Speaking is not merely a subjective act but a relational one, situated within the symbolic order and mediated by the Other.

From an objectivist perspective, speaking can be studied empirically, analyzing its neurological and physiological correlates. For example, neuroimaging can reveal the brain regions activated during speech or dialogue. From a subjectivist perspective, speaking is a means of articulating desire, constructing identity, and engaging with the Other.

In clinical practice, speaking serves as both a diagnostic tool and a therapeutic intervention. By listening to a patient's speech, the clinician gains access to their subjective world—their desires, fears, and conflicts. At the same time, the act of speaking allows the patient to externalize their experiences, making them available for reflection and transformation.

The opposition between objectivism and subjectivism must be resolved if psychiatry is to address the full complexity of the human condition. A dialectical approach offers a way forward, integrating the insights of both perspectives while avoiding their respective pitfalls. This approach acknowledges that humans are both biological and symbolic beings, shaped by interactions between the real and the symbolic, the body and language, and the material and the relational.

By embracing this dialectical framework, psychiatry can restore balance to its practices and respond to the diverse needs of patients. It can honor the insights of objectivism without reducing the subject to a mere object, and it can celebrate the contributions of subjectivism without neglecting the biological foundations of mental health.

Ultimately, the integration of objectivism and subjectivism reaffirms the centrality of the subject in psychiatry. It reminds us that the goal of psychiatric practice is not merely to alleviate symptoms but to engage with the whole person—their body, mind, and desire—and to support them in the pursuit of a meaningful and fulfilling life.

PART 6

To Resist the Death Instinct of Nothingness

An Investigation into Nothingness as the Ground of Desire

Introduction

In the final part of this book, I integrate three key aspects of the subject that, while seemingly disparate, converge on a shared focal point: **nothingness**. This void, paradoxically, not only serves as the nucleus of the subject's emergence but also sustains its continued existence. These aspects include the subject's relational dynamics, particularly in **object relations theory**—albeit reconsidered here as an **object relations theory without an object**; the **transcendental**, which underpins subjectivity and yet is marginalized in contemporary psychiatry due to its pursuit of scientific objectivity; and **mysticism**, a transcendental phenomenon aimed at returning to the nothingness from which the subject originated.

If this book were to be summarized succinctly, it could be expressed through this triptych: the subject arises from nothingness, attaches itself to the object, and shapes its relationship to that object along a transcendental path. This path relies on the mediating function of the symbol—realizing that the symbol is not equivalent to the object it signifies. As Foucault aptly noted, *"the word is not a thing"* (Foucault, 1966).

This section on mysticism will show the reverse trajectory: from the mediated relationship to the object via language back to an unmediated plunge into nothingness, where no object remains.

DOI: 10.4324/9781003675389-29

23

AN OBJECT RELATIONS THEORY WITHOUT AN OBJECT

Introduction

This text focuses on the development of object relations theory, though it acknowledges that nothingness acts as a driving force in the background. This may seem paradoxical, but it is not. Object relations theory itself emerged from nothingness. Nothingness forms the foundation of desire, which seeks its object in the Other. This section sets out the context for this perspective on object relations theory.

How Did Object Relations Theory Develop?

In psychoanalysis, a distinction exists between an interest in intrapsychic reality and external reality. The former focuses primarily on the unconscious and the conflicts that arise internally, while the latter examines the external influences shaping the structure of the subject. The external orientation is relational and object-focused, while the internal orientation is concerned with drives and their vicissitudes in relation to defenses. These divergent perspectives have deep roots in the history of psychoanalysis, with the difference of opinion between Freud and Ferenczi playing a pivotal role.

Despite the indivisibility of the subject's inside and outside, essential differences between the two perspectives continue to shape psychoanalytic focus. Overlap between inside and outside has also existed since the inception of psychoanalysis. In *Three Essays on the Theory of Sexuality*, Freud highlights how dormant passive sexual experiences become active due to

DOI: 10.4324/9781003675389-30

external influences. Freud's interest in the impact of the environment on the psyche is evident in his study of "Little Hans."

Ferenczi, however, placed greater emphasis on environmental factors in both personal development and psychoanalytic treatment. This divergence led to conflict and eventually a severance of Freud and Ferenczi's initial friendship. Freud's structural model in his second topography aligns with this connection to the external world. Karl Abraham later built on Freud's concept of the object, developing the notion of the "part object," which Melanie Klein expanded into her theory of the "good breast" and the "bad breast." Winnicott added the concept of the "transitional object," emphasizing the mother-child relationship in psychic development.

Ronald Fairbairn is considered the founder of object relations theory. Throughout his career, he refined his ideas, asserting that the events and people surrounding an individual significantly shape their internal psychological structure. The views of Klein, Winnicott, and Fairbairn align closely with Lacan's ideas regarding object relations theory. This text examines the similarities and differences between these approaches.

In 1940, Fairbairn published four articles outlining his exceptional ideas. He argued that the young child's need for relationships is central to their existence. The oral phase, rather than the Oedipal phase, was the most critical structuring stage in a child's development. Confronted by a terrifying reality, the child retreats into their inner world. For example, Fairbairn describes a child imagining that the mother's breast disappears after feeding, accompanied by the fantasy that the beloved object has been depleted. This detachment, characterized by a schizoid position, leads the child to project their fears onto the Other, distancing themselves from the engulfing mother to preserve themselves.

Fairbairn suggested that the child internalizes the bad object to safeguard the loving one. A child perceives the mother's emotional state toward them, sensing whether love and acceptance are present. This perception corresponds to an innate awareness of whole objects. If love is absent, the child withdraws, focusing solely on need satisfaction—a result of relational breakdown. Fairbairn concluded that children primarily seek a loving relationship and a sense of wholeness in the primary object. Frustration in this area gives rise to anger and hatred, which, if not channeled into development, can lead to relational collapse.

In 1944, Fairbairn published his magnum opus, *Endopsychic Structure Considered in Terms of Object-Relationships*. He argued that the libido primarily seeks an object, not drive satisfaction as Freud proposed. The internal structure of the subject emerges in relation to this object. He posited that internal structure is closely tied to external frustrations, deficiencies, or traumas, such as abuse, violence, or neglect. Unlike Klein, Fairbairn emphasized internalizing the object relationship rather than the object itself. This aligns with Lacan's idea that the subject arises from the trauma of confronting the Real, emerging through separation (castration).

It must be noted that Anglo-Saxon and Continental thought differ significantly. Anglo-Saxon approaches tend toward concreteness, often reducing the human psyche to mechanistic representations. Continental thinkers favor abstractions and transcendental constructs, recognizing the human mind's inherently transcendental nature. Psychoanalysis should remain rooted in this tradition, avoiding a "neurology of the soul." While Fairbairn stressed environmental relationships, his detailed subdivisions sometimes obscure the essence of his argument.

In the mid-20th century, structuralism emerged in France, examining the fundamental properties of culture and customs. Anthropologist Claude Lévi-Strauss pioneered this approach, drawing inspiration from Ferdinand de Saussure's linguistic theories. Thinkers such as Michel Foucault, Roland Barthes, and Jacques Lacan engaged with structuralism, acknowledging external societal structures' formative influence on the subject.

Foucault's *History of Madness* explored these themes, while Barthes deconstructed cultural phenomena such as literature, film, and fashion. Lacan applied structuralist ideas to psychoanalytic theory, particularly Freud's texts and Heidegger's philosophy. Structuralism influenced Continental philosophy and the cultural sciences, though its impact on the human sciences has been limited, partly due to the rise of biological approaches, such as Mark Solms' neuropsychoanalysis.

Lacan and the Object

Lacan's work is notoriously challenging due to his idiosyncratic language and divergence from mainstream psychoanalysis. His extensive references to philosophy, literature, and psychoanalytic texts require careful study. Key constants in his work include the hegemony of language as a structuring factor, the mirror stage, the relationship with the Other, the subject's split, and the impossibility of the Real.

Contrary to criticisms that Lacan neglects emotions, he classifies them as imaginary but devotes significant attention to transference and anxiety. Lacan's theoretical evolution remains grounded in a consistent emphasis on language's role in structuring the subject.

This text outlines the trajectory from psychoanalysis' focus on the psyche's internal structure to a relational emphasis in object relations theory. It underscores the symbolic nature of human experience and the creative potential born of nothingness. By engaging with language, psychoanalysis bridges the internal and external worlds, enabling the subject's emergence from desire and separation.

Transference

During the 1960–1961 academic year, Lacan dedicated a semester to lecturing on transference, maintaining a clear argumentative thread despite an apparently associative approach. He began by examining the asymmetry between two subjects, such as the analysand and the psychoanalyst. As an example, Lacan referred to Plato's *Symposium*, specifically the encounter between Socrates and Alcibiades.

The story is well-known: Alcibiades, a former student and lover of Socrates, disrupts a philosophical gathering on the topic of love with his drunken companions. Alcibiades declares his love for Socrates, who, uncomfortable, remains reserved and distant. In Ilja Leonard Pfeijffer's historical novel about Alcibiades, Socrates is described as "housing gods in that grotesque body." Socrates, short and unattractive, is seen by Alcibiades as possessing an internal quality—an *agalma* or ornament, a hidden treasure.

For Lacan, the *agalma* symbolizes the imperceptible quality of the Other that draws desire. This object cannot be physically observed; it is a symbolic entity expressed only in language. Alcibiades' love is directed not at a tangible object but at a symbolic absence, representing desire as a relational phenomenon without a physical basis.

Criticism of Lacan often centers on his emphasis on division, limitation, and the impossibility of the Real. Such critiques are misplaced, as these concepts are integral to Freud's foundational psychoanalytic ideas, including the rule of abstinence.

The splitting of the subject is essential for symbolization. During separation, the subject detaches from a part of itself—the Real of its body—creating a void that demands fulfilment. This void gives rise to desire, contrasting with the drive as a motivator for human expression. Language, as the primary medium of the symbolic, channels this desire. When the transition from the Real to the Symbolic fails, psychosis or personality disorders may arise. In psychosis, the Symbolic is rejected; in personality disorders, it is denied. In neurosis, excessive repression leads to symptoms charged with unconscious meaning.

Alienation also occurs within the subject as they enter the Symbolic order of language. This process distances the subject from their being, situating them "outside" themselves. By speaking, the subject simultaneously creates and reflects upon their existence, embodying the paradox of perceiving and naming from another perspective.

Objet Petit a

The object of desire, referred to as *objet petit a* (object small *a*), has no physical existence. Lacan built on Plato's *Symposium*, where Alcibiades perceives Socrates as possessing an imperceptible ornament, the *agalma*. This non-material object drives desire, embodying the creative force of nothingness.

During the separation between mother and child, both experience a shared loss, a lack of being (*manque à être*). This absence constitutes a void, propelling the subject toward symbolization. Nothingness becomes the condition for speech, as the speaking Other enables the subject's own articulation.

Symbolization and Nothingness

The subject's relationship with language involves both active and passive roles. Etymologically, "subject" derives from the Latin *subjacere* (to submit) and *subjectum* (that which is subject). The subject is simultaneously subjected to language and the bearer of its signifiers.

This duality mirrors the conscious and unconscious positions of the subject, both of which are effects of speech. Separation introduces a creative void, prompting the subject to fill this emptiness with words. The symbolic aspect of language emerges from nothingness, shaping and expressing desire.

Intermezzo: Ice Floes and Meaning

When I was about 10 years old, we went with a few boys to the park in the city. There was a small river that usually meandered quietly along its path. In the winter of 1955, it froze so hard that the river was completely frozen over in places, but here and there the water flowed so fast that ice floes were floating on it. It was a rather dangerous game for us to jump from one bank to the other via those ice floes. The trick was to reach the other side very quickly without getting wet clothes or worse. We looked like ballet dancers from Swan Lake.

The metaphor of "ice floes tapping" captures the process of meaning-making. Just as ice dancers traverse a river by briefly stepping on floating floes, the subject moves between signifiers. Meaning arises not from individual signifiers but from their interplay, much like the dancer's steps create a trajectory across the river. For Lacan, the subject exists as an effect of language, carried along by the chain of signifiers.

The metaphor of *ice tapping* also helps us understand that words never provide a complete picture of what lies beneath the surface. The sound we hear is an indication, a clue, but never the whole truth. The same goes for words: they can approximate a feeling or a thought, but they can never fully capture what the subject truly is. Words carry the subject, but they never fully reveal it.

This also explains why communication can often be so complex. One person might hear a tap on the ice and interpret it as a sign of strength, while another hears the same sound and believes the ice is fragile. Our interpretations of words differ because they resonate with our own experiences, our own "underlying waters."

Thus, *ice tapping* becomes a powerful metaphor for the use of words. It reminds us that language is not merely an instrument but also a bridge—fragile yet essential—between our inner world and that of another. It reminds us to tap carefully, to listen attentively to the sounds that return, and to respect the words we choose as carriers of something greater than themselves.

This metaphor of ice tapping can be used to determine the constellation and positioning of the subject in relation to language. The subject is then the dancer who jumps from ice floe to ice floe as a speaker says word after word. The subject is seemingly carried by the words, but in fact he comes into being in the flight from one word to the next. It is precisely in the space between the words that the subject comes to life.

Under a metonymic shift, the subject is not only a "carried" by the word but also a carrier of the chain of words.

Conclusion

In *The Ethics of Psychoanalysis*, Lacan asserts that consciousness, closely tied to speech, belongs to the symbolic rather than the natural order. Its origin lies in creation (*creatio ex nihilo*), not evolution. Desire arises from separation—between mother and child, being and symbol, and word and thing. The symbolic, lacking a material substrate, is the essence of the subject.

Psychopathology often stems from interpretative failures that manifest in symptoms or somatic complaints. Effective psychotherapy must engage with the symbolic, allowing the unspeakable to find expression through language. Physical interventions, though occasionally facilitating, often hinder this process.

This text traces psychoanalysis' evolution from an inward focus on psychic structure to an outward turn emphasizing relationality. Fairbairn's emphasis on internalizing relationships, rather than objects, resonates with Lacan's structuralist perspective. Lacan radicalized this view, linking the subject's internal structure to the Symbolic order, where the object dissolves into nothingness. This shift aligns with Continental philosophy, contrasting sharply with Anglo-Saxon objectivism.

The subject, grounded in nothingness, navigates the creative void left by separation. This dynamic demands ethical sensitivity in psychoanalytic practice, especially regarding the timing of abstinence and interpretation. Treatment strategies must consider the patient's structure, with special care for those with psychosis or limited symbolic engagement. For children, play often facilitates symbolization, allowing language and subjectivity to develop.

Ultimately, the ethical imperative in psychoanalysis is to enable speech that emerges from the abyss of nothingness, fostering creativity and the possibility of transformation.

24

PSYCHIATRY AND THE TRANSCENDENTAL

Introduction

Since the Enlightenment of the 18th century, science has distanced itself from metaphysics and the transcendental. Psychiatry, as a relatively young discipline, has largely adopted these Enlightenment ideals, focusing on empiricism and objectivity. While certain schools, such as psychoanalysis, anthropological psychiatry, and anti-psychiatry, previously offered alternative perspectives, these have been marginalized in favor of a physicalist orientation that sidelines the subject and dismisses the transcendental.

This empirical focus has led psychiatry to a theoretical impasse, where the psyche is reduced to a biological substrate that fails to capture its true nature. Psychiatry's inability to address the transcendental dimension has constrained its ability to meaningfully engage with the subject's inner life. Only by reintegrating the transcendental can psychiatry escape this reductionism and open new pathways to understanding the psyche.

The Transcendental and Psychiatry

The relationship between psychiatry and the transcendental appears contradictory: psychiatry seeks scientific legitimacy, while the transcendental is rooted in metaphysics, often dismissed as vague or speculative. However, the subjective and symbolic dimensions of mental health demand attention, as pure objectivism fails to account for the lived experience of the psyche. Science, though invaluable, cannot fully encapsulate the complexities of subjectivity, which remains central to psychiatry's mission.

DOI: 10.4324/9781003675389-31

Immanuel Kant's exploration of the transcendental in his *Critique of Pure Reason* offers insights into this dilemma. Kant defines the transcendental as knowledge concerned not with objects but with the a priori conditions that shape our perception of objects. This framework suggests that human experience is mediated by structures beyond empirical observation, such as the concept of space as a precondition for perception. Similarly, psychiatric practice must account for subjective processes that transcend the purely empirical, including language, symbolic interaction, and the intersubjective space between individuals.

Philosophers such as Edmund Husserl and Martin Heidegger expanded on the transcendental's role in human experience. Husserl's phenomenology emphasizes intentionality and perception as foundational aspects of consciousness, while Heidegger's hermeneutic phenomenology explores the existential dimensions of being. These ideas underscore the necessity of addressing the transcendental in psychiatric practice, particularly in understanding phenomena like selfhood and otherness.

Sartre's Contributions to the Transcendental

Jean-Paul Sartre, building on phenomenological traditions, offers a distinct perspective on the transcendental in his existential philosophy. In *The Transcendence of the Ego*, Sartre challenges traditional notions of the self, arguing that the ego exists outside of consciousness rather than as an intrinsic part of it. This "decentered" ego underscores the subject's dependence on external structures and the absence of a fixed foundation for selfhood.

Sartre's emphasis on "pre-reflective consciousness" highlights a state of being that precedes reflective thought, offering insights into the fluidity of the subject's experience. He further explores these ideas in *Being and Nothingness*, where he situates the subject in a space of "nothingness" that enables freedom and self-definition. For psychiatry, Sartre's work invites an exploration of the tensions between selfhood, freedom, and the existential groundlessness that shapes human existence.

Transcendental Dimensions in Psychiatry

Contemporary psychiatry has largely ignored the transcendental, favoring biological explanations for mental health conditions. However, phenomenology has seen a resurgence, offering a framework for understanding disorders such as schizophrenia. Louis Sass and Josef Parnas, for example, describe schizophrenia as a "fundamental self-disorder" marked by hyperreflexivity, which reflects a dysfunction of the transcendental structures underlying selfhood.

Additionally, methods like Open Dialogue emphasize language and interaction as central to treatment. By focusing on dialogue, this approach recognizes the symbolic and intersubjective dimensions of mental health, offering an alternative to reductionist models. Despite criticisms regarding methodological limitations, Open Dialogue highlights the potential of integrating transcendental perspectives into clinical practice.

Modern Literature on the Transcendental

Recent literature has reinvigorated the discussion of the transcendental in psychiatry. Danish psychiatrist Josef Parnas and American psychiatrist Louis Sass have been at the forefront of this movement. In *The Paradoxes of Delusion*, Sass draws on Kantian ideas to link transcendental dysfunction to psychosis, while Parnas's work explores the phenomenological disruptions of selfhood in schizophrenia. Together, they argue for a more nuanced understanding of mental disorders that incorporates subjective and transcendental dimensions.

In the Dutch-speaking world, scholars such as Gerrit Glas and Guus Labooy have explored the intersections of psychiatry, philosophy, and religion. Glas's *Fear: Experience, Structure, Power* examines existential dimensions of fear, while Labooy's *Where There Is Spirit, There Is Freedom* addresses the symbolic structuring of the psyche. Despite their religious orientations, these works emphasize the transcendental as a universal human capacity, transcending specific cultural or theological frameworks.

Mysticism as a Model of Transcendence

Mysticism provides another lens for understanding the transcendental. Mystical experiences often involve the dissolution of the ego and a direct encounter with nothingness, a state that transcends language and symbolic mediation. Figures such as Meister Eckhart and Rumi describe this process as a union with the divine, characterized by a radical surrender of selfhood.

Lacan's concept of the Real offers a psychoanalytic perspective on mysticism, framing it as an encounter with an unrepresentable dimension of experience. This confrontation with the void challenges the symbolic structures that mediate human existence, revealing the groundlessness of being. Modern psychiatry could benefit from this perspective, as it emphasizes the transformative potential of engaging with the void rather than pathologizing it.

Ethical and Practical Implications

The marginalization of the transcendental in psychiatry has significant ethical consequences. A purely physicalist approach risks dehumanizing patients by reducing them to biological entities. In contrast, a transcendental perspective emphasizes the symbolic, linguistic, and intersubjective dimensions of mental health, fostering a more compassionate and holistic approach to care.

Educational reforms are crucial to achieving this integration. Training programs for mental health professionals should include foundational concepts from phenomenology, psychoanalysis, and transcendental philosophy, emphasizing the symbolic structuring of the subject and the role of language in shaping identity. Such an approach would better equip practitioners to address the complexities of human subjectivity and the challenges of contemporary psychiatry.

Conclusion

Reintegrating the transcendental into psychiatry offers a pathway to a more nuanced and humane understanding of mental health. By embracing the symbolic and subjective dimensions of the psyche, psychiatry can move beyond its reductionist tendencies and develop a more holistic framework for treatment. Methods like Open Dialogue and insights from phenomenology and mysticism demonstrate the transformative potential of this approach, underscoring the importance of the transcendental in addressing the complexities of human existence.

25

THE ETHICAL IMPLICATIONS OF MYSTICISM AND DESIRE

Introduction

This final section seeks to weave together the intricate threads of mysticism and desire, framing them within a broader ethical and practical framework. Such an integration is essential to unlock their transformative potential for psychoanalytic praxis and modern psychiatry. Mysticism challenges conventional notions of selfhood, language, and the symbolic order. It offers a model of ethical engagement rooted in humility, creativity, and transcendence—qualities that resonate deeply with the essence of desire. Desire, as the driving force of human existence, mediates between the void of nothingness and the symbolic expressions that give life its meaning. Together, these elements invite a reimagining of how we approach the complexities of human suffering and transformation.

Ethics in the Face of Nothingness

Mysticism confronts nothingness head-on, transforming what might seem like an abyss into a fertile ground for creation and renewal. This radical engagement with nothingness is not a retreat but a courageous affirmation of life's possibilities. Ethically, this perspective challenges the defensive mechanisms that individuals and societies use to avoid uncertainty: material accumulation, ideological rigidity, and pathological adaptations. Instead, mysticism calls for an embrace of uncertainty as the foundation for authentic freedom and creativity.

DOI: 10.4324/9781003675389-32

For Lacan, the ethics of desire revolve around confronting the lack that defines human subjectivity. To desire is to acknowledge and engage with the void, articulating what cannot be fully expressed. This process is inherently ethical because it demands authenticity and a recognition of the Other. Unlike pathological attempts to disavow the void, authentic desire opens a space for symbolic expression and relationality. Such an approach reframes nothingness not as a source of despair but as the bedrock of ethical existence.

Speaking and Listening as Ethical Acts

In both mysticism and psychoanalysis, the acts of speaking and listening transcend their technical roles to become deeply ethical practices. Lacan's assertion that "the subject is the effect of speaking" underscores the transformative power of language. Through the articulation of desire, individuals navigate their inner voids and establish connections with others, creating a shared space of vulnerability and meaning-making.

Mysticism complements this idea by emphasizing the role of silence. The mystic's silence is not a withdrawal from communication but an acknowledgment of the limits of language. This mirrors the therapeutic necessity of active listening—a practice that values the symbolic expressions of the Other while accepting that full comprehension is ultimately unattainable. The therapist, like the mystic, must cultivate humility and openness, recognizing that the act of listening itself can be a transformative and ethical gesture.

The Subject in Psychiatry: Balancing Objectivity and Subjectivity

Modern psychiatry often faces a tension between its scientific foundations and the subjective realities of human experience. The mystical perspective offers a path to reconcile these opposites by emphasizing relational and transcendental dimensions of subjectivity. Rather than reducing individuals to diagnostic categories or biological mechanisms, mysticism highlights the symbolic and relational aspects that define human existence.

An ethical psychiatry would resist the tendency to treat patients as mere objects of study. Instead, it would engage with them as symbolic beings, shaped by their desires, relationships, and interactions with the Other. This approach demands a shift from rigid protocols to a more nuanced understanding of the patient as a unique individual. Such a perspective acknowledges that suffering cannot always be fully captured by empirical metrics but must also be understood through the lens of subjective experience.

Desire is often misunderstood as a problem to be solved or a source of suffering to be eradicated. Mysticism and psychoanalysis, however, reveal that desire is a vital force for growth, creativity, and connection. Mysticism teaches that fulfillment does not come from the possession of desired objects but from accepting their absence. This paradoxical realization transforms desire into a source of freedom rather than frustration.

In the therapeutic context, this understanding reshapes the role of the therapist. Instead of helping patients eliminate their symptoms, the therapist guides them to confront their desires and to tolerate the lack at the core of their being. This process fosters a transformation that is not about achieving completeness but about finding meaning and freedom in imperfection. By embracing the fragmented nature of existence, patients can reorient their desires toward more authentic and creative engagements with life.

Toward a New Praxis: Mysticism and Psychoanalysis

Both mysticism and psychoanalysis share a commitment to exploring the depths of human experience, even when it leads to discomfort or uncertainty. These disciplines challenge the notion of the self as a fixed entity, emphasizing instead its dynamic and relational nature. By integrating mystical insights into psychoanalytic praxis, therapists can develop a more holistic approach that respects the complexity of the subject.

This new praxis might include the following principles:

1. **Embracing Uncertainty:** Accepting that not all aspects of human experience can be neatly categorized or understood.
2. **Fostering Creativity:** Encouraging patients to use language, art, and other symbolic forms to express their desires and confront their fears.
3. **Valuing Silence:** Recognizing the power of silence as both a therapeutic tool and a space for reflection and transformation.
4. **Acknowledging Transcendence:** Honoring the patient's capacity for growth and transformation beyond the confines of the material and measurable.

By adopting these principles, psychoanalysis can evolve into a practice that not only addresses pathology but also nurtures the patient's potential for transcendence and renewal.

The Return to the Real: A Paradoxical Closure

As this work has explored, the subject emerges from nothingness and is sustained by the symbolic order. Mysticism represents a return to this origin—not as a retreat but as a radical affirmation of existence. In confronting the void, the mystic (and, by extension, the patient) discovers the infinite possibilities inherent in being.

This return to nothingness is not a closure but a paradoxical opening. It invites us to rethink foundational assumptions about the self, desire, and the Other. It challenges us to approach life not as a set of problems to be solved but as a mystery to be lived. This perspective transforms the void from a source of fear into a wellspring of creativity and hope.

Final Reflections

The ethical imperative of psychoanalysis and psychiatry is to keep the dialogue open—to resist the allure of definitive answers and to honor the subject's capacity for desire, transformation, and transcendence. In the face of nothingness, we do not encounter despair but the potential for infinite creativity and connection.

Mysticism reminds us that the subject is always more than the sum of their parts. By integrating its insights into psychoanalytic practice, we can reimagine these disciplines not merely as sciences but as profound arts of engagement with the human condition. In doing so, we equip ourselves to navigate the challenges of the modern world with humility, creativity, and a renewed sense of hope.

26

THE SUBJECT AS A DYNAMIC PROCESS

From Deadlock to Transformation-Symbolization as a Response to Nothingness

The emergence of the subject is intrinsically tied to their capacity for symbolization—the transformative act of giving meaning to the void left by the separation from the Real, as described by Lacan. Symbolization is not merely a response to emptiness; it is a creative endeavor that transforms absence into presence, silence into speech. By naming and signifying, the subject carves out a unique position in the symbolic order, enabling desire to be articulated. This idea echoes Heidegger's exploration of being and nothingness, where language becomes the house of Being.

The act of symbolization is foundational to both psychoanalytic practice and the broader existential project of human life. It allows individuals to weave narratives, construct identities, and establish meaningful connections with the Other. However, the symbolic is not a definitive solution to the void; rather, it acts as a bridge—a structure that facilitates the navigation of the inherent tension between being and nothingness. Julia Kristeva's theory of the semiotic and symbolic interplay illuminates this dynamic, emphasizing the oscillation between pre-verbal drives and structured language.

In therapeutic contexts, the process of symbolization can be cultivated by creating an environment where a patient's words are not merely heard but echoed, reframed, and expanded. This reflective process enables the patient to engage more deeply with their desire, confront internal limitations, and discover alternative modes of relating to themselves and others. Winnicott's concept of the "transitional space" is particularly relevant here, as it highlights the interplay between internal and external realities within a safe and facilitating environment.

DOI: 10.4324/9781003675389-33

The Dialectic of Objectivity and Subjectivity

Contemporary psychiatry's emphasis on objectivity—driven by measurable outcomes, neurobiological explanations, and replicable data—often risks neglecting the subjective dimension of human experience. While objectivist approaches offer valuable insights into the biological and structural components of mental health, they must be balanced by a recognition of the symbolic, relational, and existential aspects of the subject.

This tension between objectivity and subjectivity should not be framed as a binary opposition but as a dialectical relationship that enriches our understanding of the human condition. Objectivity, rooted in the scientific tradition, provides a framework for addressing universalizable aspects of pathology. Subjectivity, on the other hand, opens access to the lived experience, the unique narratives, and the symbolic expressions of each individual. Gadamer's hermeneutics offer a model for navigating this interplay, emphasizing the dialogical process of understanding.

The practitioner's task lies in navigating the space between scientific detachment and empathetic engagement. This dual perspective—scientific rigor combined with a deep attunement to the patient's lived world—can foster a holistic approach to care. Ricoeur's analysis of narrative identity underscores the importance of integrating these dimensions, as narratives mediate between objective facts and subjective meaning.

Desire as a Pathway to Transformation

Desire emerges as a pivotal force in the subject's engagement with the void. Rather than a static longing, desire is dynamic and generative, propelling the subject toward the Other and new possibilities of meaning. This forward motion is inherently cyclical, marked by moments of fulfillment, frustration, and renewal—a process eloquently articulated in Freud's theory of repetition compulsion and Lacan's concept of the *objet petit a*.

In therapeutic practice, desire functions as a catalyst for transformation. It motivates the patient to confront their fears, explore their unconscious resistances, and engage deeply with the therapeutic process. Simultaneously, it challenges the practitioner to remain attuned, curious, and responsive to the evolving needs of the patient. Here, the transformative potential of language becomes evident. Lacan's assertion that "the subject is the effect of speaking" highlights the power of articulation in shaping identity and fostering change.

This dynamic is not confined to the therapeutic encounter. In everyday life, the act of speaking—whether through conversation, writing, or artistic expression—allows the subject to reframe experiences, articulate desires, and envision new futures. The work of Viktor Frankl, particularly his emphasis on meaning-making in the face of suffering, resonates with this perspective, demonstrating how desire and language intertwine in the pursuit of transformation.

The Role of Ethics in Practice

The ethical foundation of psychoanalysis and psychiatry rests on their commitment to the subject's dignity, freedom, and autonomy. This ethical stance requires a respect for the subject's unique trajectory and a willingness to engage with the ambiguity and complexity of human existence. Emmanuel Levinas's philosophy of the Other provides a compelling framework for understanding this commitment, emphasizing the primacy of ethical responsibility in human relationships.

In practice, this ethical orientation manifests in various ways: through attentive listening, sensitivity to symbolic expressions, and a commitment to fostering conditions that allow the subject to articulate their desires. It requires practitioners to strike a delicate balance between presence and absence, guidance and restraint, and empathy and detachment. This balance echoes Bion's concept of "containing" the patient's experience while allowing space for their growth and transformation.

Crucially, the ethical imperative in psychoanalysis is not to impose meaning but to facilitate its emergence. By holding space for the subject's voice, the practitioner helps transform the void of nothingness into a source of creativity and potential. This process aligns with Derrida's notion of deconstruction, where meaning emerges through the interplay of presence and absence, opening new pathways for understanding.

The Mystical Dimension: Returning to the Void

Mystical traditions offer profound insights into the subject's relationship with nothingness. Across various spiritual systems—from Christian mysticism to Zen Buddhism—there is a recurring theme of dissolving the self to encounter the ultimate Other. This dissolution is not experienced as annihilation but as a return to the origin, where separations are transcended, and unity is found.

Psychoanalysis mirrors this mystical journey when the subject confronts the limitations of their symbolic structures. By acknowledging the void at the heart of their being, the subject can relinquish rigid identifications and embrace a more fluid, dynamic sense of self. The writings of Rumi and Meister Eckhart illustrate this cyclical confrontation with the void as a source of renewal and transcendence.

Rather than an escape from reality, this mystical engagement with the void represents a deeper encounter with it. It challenges the subject to embrace ambiguity, accept uncertainty, and find meaning amid the tensions of existence. As Kristeva notes in *Black Sun*, such encounters with emptiness can be profoundly transformative, enabling the subject to reconstruct meaning from the ruins of despair.

Toward a New Vision of the Subject

This chapter has explored the complexities of the subject, tracing its emergence from the symbolic order to its engagement with desire, language, and the Other. We have argued that the subject is not a fixed entity but a dynamic process shaped by its encounters with nothingness and its capacity for symbolization. This vision challenges reductionist paradigms, affirming the materiality of the body, the reality of the symbolic, and the transcendental dimensions of human existence.

By resisting the deadlock of nothingness, we affirm the subject's potential for creativity, connection, and transformation. By embracing the tensions and contradictions of human life, we open new pathways for understanding and healing. And by holding space for the subject's voice, we honor the dignity and complexity of the human condition.

Through this lens, we envision a psychoanalysis and psychiatry that are scientifically rigorous, ethically grounded, and profoundly attuned to the depths of human experience. Such an approach not only addresses suffering but also fosters growth, offering the subject new possibilities for living meaningfully in the face of life's inevitable uncertainties.

27

EVERYTHING OR NOTHING

About Mysticism and the Genesis of the Subject

Introduction

What should one do with a writer about mystical experience if he lacks that experience? Does this thinker have the right to speak about it? I am one of those outsiders who—as far as I am aware—has not had any mystical experience. Yet there are holes in this reasoning when one considers that there are phenomena very similar to, and perhaps overlapping with, mystical experiences that people without such contact, i.e., outsiders, may also encounter. I am thinking of having dreams, orgasms, psychoses, and experiencing music. This is perhaps more the case with the latter three than with dreams because imagination still plays a role there. To understand this, I must delve deeper into the matter, which touches on the structural relationship between the symbolic system of language and the Real, where language is excluded, and there is immediacy—the circumstance that the mystic aims at (Foucault, 1966; Lacan, 1994).

This text revolves around the theme of *nothingness*, the focal point of mystical experience. In my journey through *The Cloud of Unknowing*, as an anonymous writer from the 14th century so aptly described mysticism, I have been guided by both mystics and thinkers about mysticism and allowed my own pseudo-mystical experiences to resonate with me. I was also guided by the relevant texts of Marc De Kesel. In this exploration, the similarities and differences between mystical experiences and psychosis are discussed.

DOI: 10.4324/9781003675389-34

Nothingness as the Beginning and Endpoint

Life begins in nothingness and ends in nothingness. In between, life unfolds in phases of development, events, adventures if you will, decline, and death. Amid this kaleidoscope of experiences, the subject emerges with a certain structure, highly dependent on the environment in which it manifests itself. Speculations about the prenatal period abound, but what the fetus experiences depends on interpretations by researchers and the person in question. Whether something is perceived during the fetal phase is hard to determine, as the future person cannot later communicate anything about it due to the absence of language faculty during that phase—the faculty that enables transferability and self-awareness.

It is likely that perceptual processes occur during pregnancy and leave traces in the neural network. It is also conceivable that fetal-phase experiences resurface later in life as associations with nirvana. It is not without significance that we connect nothingness with eternity and rest. It is also understandable that mystics seek this nothingness. Nothingness is often equated with God, as can be read in Meister Eckhart (Eckhart, 2017).

Mysticism is in vogue, not only among the religious in Western society and other cultures but also among atheist groups who call themselves followers of "modern spirituality." Mysticism is a substantial part of Zen Buddhism, the Sufi movement among Muslims, the Advaita Vedanta of Hindus, and Jewish Kabbalists. Even atheist thinkers such as Martin Heidegger and Jean-Paul Sartre were intrigued by Meister Eckhart's speculative philosophy.

According to Meister Eckhart, God is not a living being; God is being itself. What we usually understand as God involves human attributions that devalue the essence of God. God cannot be known and, therefore, falls outside the symbolic system. God is what religious mystics aim for in their search.

Descartes' Selfie

Descartes also sought the foundation of science but found no freedom to do so in 17th-century France and moved to the more tolerant Netherlands. The Netherlands of those days was a haven of freedom, though not entirely. Freethinkers like Spinoza were expelled from their communities for views like equating God with nature (*deus sive natura*).

Descartes found the conditions to think freely but left his faith in God intact. He even located its basis in the pineal gland (*epiphysis*), through which humans maintained contact with the supernatural and the relationship between body and mind. This Cartesian salvage operation for God contrasts sharply with his analysis of knowledge acquisition.

Consulting himself, Descartes took a relentless "selfie" of this process, questioning everything. Finally, he concluded that while he could doubt everything, he could not doubt the act of doubting itself. This act led him to himself, the thinking subject. Thus, doubting and thinking gained ontological status: "I think, therefore I am" (*je pense, donc je suis*).

This cogito fundamentally altered philosophy: theocentric thinking gave way to homocentric thinking, centering on the subject. This shift replaced the theocentric constellation with a focus on the subject, initiating far-reaching consequences in Western culture.

The Goal Is Never Achieved

When we attempt to capture an object in words, we face an insurmountable difficulty. Many objects can be perceived, but that is all. Some objects require resources like microscopes or particle accelerators for perception. Others, such as virtual objects, exist only in theory or fantasy.

Language lets us conjure non-existent things, such as devils, angels, God, and nothingness. This ability to symbolically manifest the non-existent is unique to humans and central to language's symbolic capacity. While this capacity fosters creativity, it can also lead to fake news and conspiracy theories.

To achieve the mystical experience, the mystic must bypass the symbolic system and thus arrive at nothingness or *das Ding an sich*. This journey parallels that of psychosis.

Mysticism and the Self

Mystics search for the essence of the self, the ground of being, often ending in nothingness. They miss their target and vanish into thin air. Mysticism reveals that the self is neither inside nor outside the subject but a boundary phenomenon between the two. The self resides in this liminal space, metaphorically represented by the skin.

The self is thus not a location but a phenomenon in the trajectory from outside to inside. Through perception, the outside moves inward. Language, which mediates between these realms, shapes the subject. Mysticism, then, must be situated in this boundary-crossing space, where it explores the void.

A Plea for Mysticism

Mysticism and psychosis, inherent to human existence, must be taken seriously by the human sciences. Dismissing them as mere aberrations or brain diseases reflects the reductionist biologism dominating science today. Structural psychoanalysis offers a counterbalance, allowing the unconscious to speak and illuminate the darkness of nothingness.

Mystical experiences, though risky, foster profound insights into the human condition. Research into mysticism, like its practice, requires an openness to uncharted intellectual and experiential territories.

The Mystical Experience as Psychotic Guided Fantasy

Psychosis is regarded in psychiatry as one of the most severe mental states. Psychotic patients may experience hallucinations, delusions, or strange perceptions of their own bodies. These experiences are usually involuntary and accompanied by fear and severe discomfort. Psychotic patients with grandiose ideas are particularly challenging for their families and surroundings. A hallmark of psychosis is the loss of contact with reality.

As previously mentioned, the mystical experience parallels psychosis in its potential for losing touch with reality. The key difference is that mystical experience is voluntary, conscious, and usually controlled. However, even this can sometimes go wrong. The mystic must know the way back to reality to safely return to the symbolic order.

The question remains: why does the mystic willingly enter such a potentially dangerous state? For the religious mystic, it is a means of coming closer to God or even uniting with Him, which often carries narcissistic motives. For the non-religious mystic, the quest might initially seem unrelated to faith. Instead, the motivation may lie in a desire to coincide with the Real—a space that is not necessarily pleasant. Letting go of the symbolic shield of language exposes the mystic to raw, unfamiliar perceptions, often accompanied by disintegration or a sense of eternal falling.

The journey of the mystic is difficult and perilous. Adequate preparation is essential. The bliss of achieving the mystical goal often comes with bitter aftereffects, akin to the ambivalence of *jouissance*.

Positive Mysticism

Contrary to radical views on nothingness, many mystics find positive outcomes in their pursuit. Something positive can emerge from nothingness. Thinkers like Schopenhauer and Schelling (Lütkehaus, 2008), and arguably Lacan, reflect this idea.

For the most radical mystics, humans originate in nothingness and return to it upon death. For them, death is the ultimate teacher and a mystical practice in itself (Lütkehaus).

On the other hand, radical nihilists such as Nietzsche, Louis Aragon, and possibly Juan de la Cruz, fail to discover anything positive in mysticism. Juan de la Cruz, even after ascending the summit of Mount Carmel of the Perfect Spirit, encounters only "nada" (nothingness) sevenfold.

The Creative Nothingness

Hegel offers a positive reinterpretation of nothingness in his dialectical logic: *Being + Nothingness = Becoming.*

If we assert that nothingness only leads to more nothingness, the question arises: what then of life? Even if life emerges from nothingness, it still generates meaning and value before returning to its origin. Heidegger suggests in *The Principle of Ground* that all things have a ground, even if that ground ultimately collapses into nothingness. In Hegel, being and nothingness interweave dialectically, producing a creative interplay.

While linear reasoning suggests that being stems from nothing in a straightforward progression, Žižek's interpretation of Hegel hints at a more nuanced dialectic: a simultaneous concurrence of being, nothingness, and becoming.

Desire and speaking emerge from the void of separation and alienation. Every spoken word pierces the Real, leaving behind the residue of meaning. Through this process, the subject emerges. The subject, as Lacan posits, is the effect of speaking.

Following Lacan, the subject's core is void. Seeking this core is itself a mystical act, one that many avoid due to fear of confronting the emptiness. Instead, the subject fills this void with stories and language. Mystical exploration of this void may appear unnatural, as it seeks to confront what most avoid.

Damasio, by contrast, sees this void as filled with neurons, synapses, and neurotransmitters. His perspective diverges sharply from the one presented here, effectively turning back the clock on Western thought by centuries.

Mysticism and the Contemporary World

Since the 1960s, society has shifted toward inward introspection, with diminishing connection to others. This disconnection fosters terrorism, drug use, and an autistic-like retreat into self-gratification, mysticism, and escapism. Mysticism may now reflect resistance to an overly materialistic, data-driven world that fosters unease and saturation.

This mysticism, however, is distinct from traditional forms. It is often divorced from organized religion or collective spiritual practices, reflecting instead an individualistic pursuit of transcendence.

Overview

Western culture periodically gravitates toward the idea of nothingness, from Parmenides through Hamlet to Heidegger, and now Žižek's *Less Than Nothing*. Mystics, nihilists, philosophers, and seekers explore nothingness for various reasons, ranging from the search for God to the exploration of ethical groundlessness or resistance to materialism.

Mystics seek God, but may not always find Him. Nihilists and philosophers, by contrast, explore the inherent emptiness or absurdity of existence. The increasing interest in mysticism today reveals a deep-seated desire for the transcendental amid a materialistic world.

At the intersection of mysticism and psychosis lies the subject's precarious balance between "everything" and "nothing." Mystics consciously seek the void, while psychotics are involuntarily thrust into it. Both confront the same fundamental question of existence: "Who am I?"

BIBLIOGRAPHY

Abraham, Karl. 1923. *Versuch Einer Entwicklungsgeschichte Der Libido Auf Grund Der Psychoanalyse Seelischer Störungen - Neue Arbeiten Zur Ärztlichen Psychoanalyse Heft II*. Frankfurt am Main: Fischer Verlag.

Achterhuis, Hans. 2021. *Geloof in Geweld* [Belief in Violence]. Rotterdam: Lemniscaat.

American Psychiatric Association. 2016. *Diagnostic and Statistical Manual of Mental Disorders (DSM-5)*. Washington, DC: APA.

Anderson, C. A., and C. M. Filley. 2016. "Delusional Misidentification Syndromes: Progress and New Challenges." *The Journal of Neuropsychiatry and Clinical Neurosciences* 8 (3): 160–161.

Anonymous. (Late 14th century). *The Cloud of Unknowing*. Internet: Full audiobook.

Apuleius, Lucius. (n.d.) *Metamorphoses*. Internet: Brill Scholar Editions, Apuleius Online, 125–175.

Arendt, Hannah. 1971, 1979. *The Life of the Mind. Volume Two: Willing*. San Diego: Harcourt Trade Publishers.

Atta, K., N. Forlenza, M. Gujski, S. Hashmi, and G. Isaac. 2006. "Delusional Misidentification Syndromes: Separate Disorders or Unusual Presentations of Existing DSM-IV Categories?" *Psychiatry* 3 (9): 56–61.

Aulagnier, Piera. 2009. *Dossier Wolfson en l'Affaire du "Schizo et les Langues."* Paris: Gallimard.

Badiou, Alain. 2006. *L'être et l'événement*. Paris: Éditions du Seuil.

Bakhtin, M. M. 1929, 1978. *Le Marxisme et la Philosophie du Langage: Essai d'Application de la Méthode Sociologique en Linguistique*. Paris: Les Éditions de Minuit.

Bakhtin, M. M. 1993. *Towards a Philosophy of the Act*. Edited by Vadim Liapinov and Michael Holquist. Translated by Vadim Liapinov. Austin: University of Texas Press.

Bally, Charles, and Albert Sechehaye. 1916, 1981. "Préface de la Première Édition." In *Cours de Linguistique Générale de Ferdinand de Saussure*. Paris: Payot.

Barahona, Rodrigo. 2025. *Negative Hallucinosis in Wilfred Bion's Theory of Transformations: On Finding One's Ghost*. London and New York: Routledge.
Barthes, Roland. 1953, 1972. *Le Degré Zéro de l'Écriture*. Paris: Éditions du Seuil, Points.
Barthes, Roland. 1975. *Roland Barthes par Roland Barthes*. Paris: Éditions du Seuil.
Barthes, Roland. 2010. *Roland Barthes by Roland Barthes*. New York: Hill and Wang Editors.
Bateson, Gregory. 1956, 1978. *Steps to an Ecology of Mind*. London, Toronto, Sydney, New York: Paladin Granada Publishing.
Bateson, Gregory, Donald D. Jackson, Jay Haley, and John H. Weakland. 1956. "Towards a Theory of Schizophrenia." *Behavioral Science* 1 (4): 251–264.
Bergson, Henri. 1889, 2001. *Time and Free Will: An Essay on the Immediate Data of Consciousness*. Garden City, NY: Dover Publications.
Bergson, Henri. 1906, 1998. *Creative Evolution*. New York: Dover Publications, Inc.
Berrios, German E. 1996. *The History of Mental Symptoms*. Cambridge: Cambridge University Press.
Bion, Wilfred R. 1965. *Transformations*. London: Heinemann.
Bleuler, Eugen. 1919. *Das Autistisch-Undiziplinierte Denken in der Medizin und Seine Überwindung*. Berlin: Verlag von Julius Springer.
Blom, Jan Dirk. 2010. *A Dictionary of Hallucinations*. New York, Dordrecht, Heidelberg, London: Springer.
Bonnefoi, C. 1966. "L'homme est-il Mort? Un Entretien avec Michel Foucault." *Ars et Loisirs* 38: 8.
Braam, Arjan W., Dorly J. H. Deeg, Theo G. van Tilburg, A. T. F. Beekman, and Willem van Tilburg. 1998. "Gerotranscendentie als Levensperspectief: Een Eerste Empirische Benadering bij Ouderen in Nederland." *Tijdschrift voor Gerontologie en Geriatrie* 29: 24–32.
Brakel, Linda A. 1989. "Understanding Negative Hallucination: Toward a Developmental Classification of Disturbances in Reality Awareness." *Journal of the American Psychoanalytic Association* 37 (2): 437–463.
Breuer, J. & Freud, S. (1893–1895). Fraulein Anna O. Case Histories from Studies on Hysteria. In J. Strachey (Ed. & Trans.), *Standard Edition of the Complete Psychological Works of Sigmund Freud* (Vol. II, pp. 19–47). London: Hogarth Press.
Calmeyn, Marc. 2011. "Transparantie en Transcendentie: Over Zichtbaarheid en Onzichtbaarheid in de Biologische Psychiatrie." *Collationes* 41 (4): 409–420. Accessed December 2023. https://marccalmeyn.be/images/bibliografie/artikels/collationesCalmeyn.pdf
Capgras, Jean, and J. Rebcul-Lachaaux. 1923. "L'Illusion des 'Sosies' dans un Délire Systématisé Chronique." *Société Clinique de Médecine Mentale* 11: 6–16.
Chalmers, David J. 1996. *The Conscious Mind: In Search of a Fundamental Theory*. New York-Oxford: Oxford University Press.
Chalmers, David J. 2022. *Reality+: Virtual Worlds and the Problems of Philosophy*. Rushden: Allen Lane, Penguin Books.
Christodoulou, George N., Margarita Margariti, and Nicholas Christodoulou. 2018. "Delusional Misidentifications in a Procrustean Bed." *Psichiatriki* 29 (1): 15–18.
Churchland, Patricia. 1981. "Eliminative Materialism and the Propositional Attitudes." *Journal of Philosophy* 78: 67–90.

Clérambault, Gaëtan Gatian de. 1942. *Œuvre Psychiatrique I–II*. Paris: Presses Universitaires de France.
Cotard, Jules. 1884. "L'Origine Psychomotrice du Délire." Edited by J. Faret (1891). *Congrès International de Médecine Mentale*.
Couturat, Louis. 1903. *Opuscules et Fragments Inédits de Leibniz*. Paris: Félix Alcan.
Craft, Robert. 1972. *Stravinsky: The Chronicle of a Friendship 1948–1971*. London: Victor Gollancz.
Damasio, Antonio R. 1994. *Descartes' Error*. New York: Evans Books.
Damasio, Antonio R. 1999. *The Feeling of What Happens*. London: Mariner Books, Harper Collins.
Darby, Ryan R., Sebastien Laganiere, Alvaro Pascual-Leone, S. Prasad, and Michael D. Fox. 2007. "Finding the Imposter: Brain Connectivity of Lesions Causing Delusional Misidentifications." *Brain* 140 (2): 497–507.
De Kesel, Marc. 2012. *Žižek*. Amsterdam-Leuven: Boom-LannooCampus.
De Kesel, Marc. 2019. *Het Münchhausenparadigma: Waarom Freud en Lacan Ertoe Doen*. Nijmegen: Vantilt Uitgeverij.
De Kesel, Marc A. B. M. 2021. *Ik, God en Mezelf: Mystiek als Deconstructie*. Amsterdam: Sjibbolet.
De Kesel, Marc A. B. M. 2023. *Effacing the Self*. New York: SUNY Press.
De Vleminck, J. 2020. "Obstakels of Kwintessens? Sándor Ferenczi over de Tegenoverdracht." *Tijdschrift voor Psychoanalyse en haar Toepassingen* 27 (4): 273–286.
Dennett, Daniel. 1991, 1993. *Consciousness Explained*. London: Penguin Books.
Derrida, Jacques. 1967. *De la Grammatologie*. Paris: Éditions de Minuit.
Descartes, René. 1637, 1937. Discours de la Méthode. In *Descartes Oeuvres Lettres*. Paris: La Pléiade.
Dörner, Klaus, and Ursula Plog. 1983, 2015. *Irren ist Menschlich: Lehrbuch der Psychiatrie und Psychotherapie*. Köln: Psychiatrie Verlag.
Dostoevsky, Fyodor M. 1846. *The Double*. Internet Archive.
Eckhart, Meister Johannes. 2017. *Mystische Schriften*. Musaicum Books. Kindle Edition, internet.
Engel, George. 1977. "The Need for a New Medical Model: A Challenge for Biomedicine." *Science* 196 (4286): 129–136.
Ettinger, Bracha L. 2006. *The Matrixial Borderspace*. Minneapolis: University of Minnesota Press.
Evans, Dylan. 1996. *An Introductory Dictionary of Lacanian Psychoanalysis*. London-New York: Routledge.
Ey, Henri. 1938, 1975. *Des Idées de Jackson à un Modèle Organo-Dynamique en Psychiatrie*. Paris: Privat.
Fairbairn, William R. D. 1944, 2013. "Endopsychic Structure Considered in Terms of Object-Relationships." In *The Writings of Melanie Klein Volume IV*, 224–225. London: Routledge.
Fairbairn, William R. D. 1963. "Synopsis of an Object-Relations Theory of the Personality." *The International Journal of Psychoanalysis* 44: 224–225.
Feyaerts, J., M. G. Hendriksen, S. Vanheule, I. Myin-Germeys, and L. A. Sass. 2021a. "Delusions Beyond Beliefs: A Critical Overview of Diagnostic, Aetiological, and Therapeutic Schizophrenia Research from a Clinical-Phenomenological Perspective." *The Lancet Psychiatry* 8: 237–249.
Feyaerts, J., W. Kusters, and Z. van Duppen. 2021b. "Uncovering the Realities of Delusional Experience in Schizophrenia: A Qualitative Phenomenological Study in Belgium." *The Lancet Psychiatry* 8: 784–796.

Foucault, Michel. 1961. *Madness and Civilization*. Accessed online. Vintage Books.

Foucault, Michel. 1963. *The Birth of the Clinic: An Archaeology of Medical Perception*. Accessed online. Vintage Books.

Foucault, Michel. 1966. *The Archaeology of Knowledge*. Accessed online. Vintage Books.

Foucault, Michel. 1966, 2002. *The Order of Things: An Archaeology of the Human Sciences*. London: Routledge.

Foucault, Michel. 1969, 2002. *The Archaeology of Kwowledge*. (Trans. A.M. Sheridan Smith. London/New York: Routledge.

Freud, Sigmund. 1890. Psychical (or Mental) Treatment. In J. Strachey (Ed. & Trans.), *The Standard Edition of the Complete Psychological Works of Sigmund Freud* (Vol. 7, pp. 281–302). London: Hogarth Press.

Freud, Sigmund. 1895, 1950. Project for a Scientific Psychology. In *The Standard Edition of the Complete Psychological Works of Sigmund Freud*, Vol. 1: 295–343. London: Hogarth Press.

Freud, Sigmund. 1911. "Psycho-Analytic Notes Upon an Autobiographical Account of a Case of Paranoia." *The Standard Edition of the Complete Psychological Works of Sigmund Freud*, Vol. 12. London: Hogarth Press.

Freud, Sigmund. 1914. "On Narcissism: An Introduction." *The Standard Edition of the Complete Psychological Works of Sigmund Freud*, Vol. 14. London: Hogarth Press.

Freud, Sigmund. 1915. "Instincts and Their Vicissitudes." In J. Strachey (Ed. and Trans.) *The Standard Edition of the Complete Psychological Works of Sigmund Freud*, Vol. 14, pp. 109–140. London: Hogarth Press.

Freud, Sigmund. 1919. "The Uncanny." *The Standard Edition of the Complete Psychological Works of Sigmund Freud*, Vol. 17. London: Hogarth Press.

Freud, Sigmund. 1922. "Some Neurotic Mechanisms in Jealousy, Paranoia, and Homosexuality." *The Standard Edition of the Complete Psychological Works of Sigmund Freud*, Vol. 18. London: Hogarth Press.

Freud, Sigmund. 1923. "The Ego and the Id and Other Works." *The Standard Edition of the Complete Psychological Works of Sigmund Freud*, Vol. 19. London: Hogarth Press.

Freud, Sigmund. 1925. "An Autobiographical Study." *The Standard Edition of the Complete Psychological Works of Sigmund Freud*, Vol. 20: 1–74. London: Hogarth Press.

Fromm, Erich. 1941, 2001. *The Fear of Freedom*. London: Routledge.

Gerritse, Frank. 2019. "Open Vragen Rondom Open Dialogue." Accessed online. https://dejongepsychiater.nl

Glas, Gerrit. 1991. *Concepten van Angst en Angststoornissen*. Amsterdam/Lisse: Swets & Zeitlinger B.V.

Glas, Gerrit. 2001. *Angst: Beleving, Structuur en Macht*. Amsterdam: Boom.

Green, André. 1993, 2011. *The Work of the Negative*. London-New York: Routledge.

Hamburger, Martijn. 2020. "Fairbairns Interne Saboteur 75 Jaar Later." *Tijdschrift voor Psychoanalyse & haar Toepassingen* 27 (4): 248–260.

Hazif-Thomas, Claude. 2016. "Psychose, Mélancholie et Hallucinations Négatives chez le Sujet Âgé." *Annales Médico-Psychologiques, Revue Psychiatrique* 174 (3): 185–188.

Hazif-Thomas, Claude, François Stephan, Marie Walter, and Philippe Thomas. 2014. "Hallucination Négative, Conscience de Soi et Avancée en Âgé." *L'Encéphale* 41 (2): 168–173.

Hegel, Georg Wilhelm Friedrich. 1807, 1979. *Phenomenology of Spirit*. Oxford: Oxford University Press.

Heidegger, Martin. 1927, 2008. *Being and Time*. Glasgow: HarperCollins Publishers.
Heidegger, Martin. 1929, 1998. *What is Metaphysics*. Cambridge: Cambridge University Press.
Heidegger, Martin. 1955–1956. *Der Satz von Grund*. Stuttgart: Klett-Cotta.
Heidegger, Martin. 1956, 1974. The Principle of Ground. *Man and World* 7: 207–222. https://doi.org/10.1007/BF01248755
Heisenberg, Werner. 1958, 2000. *Physics and Philosophy*. New York: Penguin Books.
Hinshelwood, Robert D., and Wilhelm Skogstad. 2000. *Observing Organisations: Anxiety, Defence and Culture in Health Care*. London: Routledge.
Hoffmann, Ernst Theodor Amadeus. 1815, 2007. *The Devil's Elixir*. London: Grosvenor House Publishing.
Horst Van Der, Louis. 1946. *Anthropologische Psychiatrie*. Amsterdam: Van Holkeman & Warendorf N.V.
Husserl, Edmund. 1937. *The Crisis in European Sciences and Transcendental Phenomenology*. Translated by David Carr. Evanston, IL: Northwestern University Press.
Husserl, Edmund. 1937, 2018. *De Crisis van de Europese Wetenschappen en de Transcendentale Fenomenologie*. Amsterdam: Boom.
Huxley, Aldous. 1954, 2009. *The Doors of Perception*. London: Harper Torch.
Jackson, John Hughlings. 1884. "The Croonian Lectures on Evolution and Dissolution of the Nervous System." *British Medical Journal* 1: 591–593.
Jaspers, Karl. 1913. *Allgemeine Psychopathologie*. Berlin-Heidelberg: Springer Verlag.
Johnston, Adrian. (2018). *A New German Idealism: Hegel, Žižek, and Dialectical Materialism*. Columbia University Press.
Jonghe, F. de, and O. Markx. 1979a. "Het Verschijnsel van Capgras: Over 'L'Illusion des Sosies'." *Tijdschrift voor P.sychiatrie* 21 (1): 600–615.
Jonghe, F. de, and O. Markx. 1979b. "Misidentificatie: Over het Foutief Identificeren van Personen." *Tijdschrift voor Psychiatrie* 21 (1): 583–599.
Joseph, Andrew B. 1994. "Observations on the Epidemiology of the Delusional Misidentification Syndromes in the Boston Metropolitan Area (1983–1984)." *Psychology* 27: 150–153.
Kalinova, Milena. 2018. "Exotopy: Mikhail Bakhtin and Jacques Lacan on the Outside Context of Discourse." *Slavica Tergestina: European Slavic Studies Journal* 20 (1): 98–117.
Kandel, Eric. 2018, 2019. *The Disordered Mind*. New York: Farrar, Straus and Giroux.
Kant, Immanuel. 1788, 1998. *Critique of Pure Reason*. Translated by Paul Guyer and Allen W. Wood. Cambridge: Cambridge University Press.
Kant, Immanuel. 1781, 2004. *Kritiek van de Zuivere Rede*. Amsterdam: Boom.
Karskens, Machiel. 1986. *Waarheid als Macht: Een Onderzoek naar de Filosofische Ontwikkeling van Michel Foucault*. Nijmegen: Stichting Te Elfder Ure.
Kim, Jaegwon. 1993. *Supervenience and Mind*. Cambridge: Cambridge University Press.
Klein, Melanie. 1984. *Narrative of a Child Analysis: The Writings of Melanie Klein, Volume IV*. New York: The Free Press.
Koehler, B., Silver, A.-L., and Karon, B. 2013. "Psychodynamic Approaches to Understanding Psychosis: Defenses Against Terror." In *Models of Madness: Psychological, Social and Biological Approaches to Psychosis*, edited by John Read and Jacqui Dillon, 238–248. London: Routledge.
Kopland, Rutger. 1972. "Wie wat vindt heeft slecht gezocht." In *Vier Gedichten*. Amsterdam: G.A. van Oorschot.

Kraepelin, Emil. 1904. *Psychiatrie: Ein Lehrbuch für Studirende und Ärzte*. 7th ed. Leipzig: Verlag von Johann Ambrosius Barth.
Kroon, Jos de. 1993. *Taal en Psychose (Language and Psychosis): Een Onderzoek naar de Relatie tussen Taal en Psychose volgens het Structuralisme van Jacques Lacan en een Mogelijke Psychotherapie*. Utrecht: Uitgeverij De Tijdsstroom.
Kroon, Jos de. 2004. *Schizofrenie Tussen Symptoom en Subject (Schizophrenia Between Symptom and Subject): Een Archeologie van de Psychose*. Antwerpen-Apeldoorn: Garant.
Kroon, Jos de. 2005. "Jouissance a Cinque Voci: Muziek en het Onmogelijke Genieten." *Tijdschrift voor Psychoanalyse* 11 (2): 98–108.
Kroon, Jos de. 2010. *De Stem van de Ander: Over (Verbale) Hallucinaties (The Voice of the Other: On (Verbal) Hallucinations)*. Antwerpen-Apeldoorn: Garant-Uitgevers.
Kroon, Jos de, and Thiery Verplancke. 2017. "Als in een Zwarte Spiegel: Over het Syndroom van Cotard." ("As in a Black Mirror: On Cotard's Syndrom"). *Tijdschrift voor Psychoanalyse* 23 (4): 105–115.
Kusters, Wouter. 2020. *A Philosophy of Madness: The Experience of Psychotic Thinking*. Cambridge, MA: MIT Press.
Kwant, Remi C. 1978. *Structuralisten en Structuralisme*. Alphen aan den Rijn: Samsom Uitgeverij.
Lacan, Jacques. 1949, 2006. The Mirror Stage as Formative of the Function of the I as Rdvealed in Psychoanalytic Experience. In B. Fink (Trans.), *Ecrits: The First Complete Edition in English*. New York/London: W.W. Norton & Company. (orig. presented in 1949 as *Le stade du moroir comme formateur de la fonction du Je*.
Lacan, Jacques. 2019 (1958–1959). *The Seminar of Jacques Lacan, Book VI: Desire and its Interpretation*. Edited by Jacques-Alain Miller, translated by Bruce Fink. Cambridge: Polity Press.
Lacan, Jacques. 1964, 1977b. *The Seminar of Jacques Lacan: Book XI, The Four Fundamental Concepts of Psychoanalysis*. Translated by Alan Sheridan. London: Hogarth Press.
Lacan, Jacques. 1966. *Écrits*. Paris: Éditions du Seuil.
Lacan, Jacques. 1975. *The Seminar of Jacques Lacan: Book XX, Encore*. Edited by Jacques-Alain Miller. Paris: Éditions du Seuil.
Lacan, Jacques. 1977. *Écrits: A Selection*. Translated by Alan Sheridan. London: Tavistock.
Lacan, Jacques. 1986, 1992. *The Seminar of Jacques Lacan: Book VII, The Ethics of Psychoanalysis*. Edited by Jacques-Alain Miller. Translated by Dennis Porter. New York: W.W. Norton & Company.
Lacan, Jacques. 1994. *The Seminar of Jacques Lacan: Book IV, The Object Relation*. Edited by Jacques-Alain Miller. Translated by Adrian Price. Cambridge: Polity Press.
Lacan, Jacques. 1994. The Name-of-the-Father. In A. Sheridan (Trans.), *The Four Fundamental Concepts of Psycho-Analysis*. London: W.W. Norton & Company.u8
Lacan, Jacques. 2004. *The Seminar of Jacques Lacan: Book X, Anxiety*. Edited by Jacques-Alain Miller. Translated by Adrian Price. Toronto: John Wiley & Sons.
Lamettrie, Julien Offray de. 1748, 1995. *Man a Machine*. Accessed online.
Leibniz, Gottfried Wilhelm. 1686, 1981. *Discourse on Metaphysics*. Translated by Machiel Karskens. Bussum: Het Wereldvenster.
Lévi-Strauss, Cl. 1962. *La pensée sauvage*. Paris: Plon.
Lévi-Strauss, Cl. 1973, 1977. *Structural Anthropology*. London: Penguin Books.

Libet, Benjamin, Curtis A. Glaeson, Elwood W. Wright, and Dennis K. Pearl. 1983. "Time of Conscious Intention to Act in Relation to Onset of Cerebral Activity (Readiness-Potential)." *Brain* 106: 623–642.

Loo, Danielle T. M. van de, Noor Saämena, Peter Janse, Martijn van Vliet, and A. W. Braam. 2022. "De Waardering van de Zes Dimensies van Positieve Gezondheid in de GGZ." *Tijdschrift voor Psychiatrie* 64: 87–93.

Lütkehaus, Ludger. 2003, 2008. *Nichts: Abschied von Sein. Ende der Angst.* Frankfurt am Main: Haffmans Verlag.

Mahler, Margaret S., Fred Pine, and Anni Bergman. 1975. *The Psychological Birth of the Human Infant*. New York: Basic Books.

Mauss, Marcel. 1923–1924, 2017. *The Gift*. London: Routledge.

Meltzer, Donald & Anna Sabatini Scolmati. 2009. Psychotic Illness in Early Childhood: Ten Years on from Explorations in Autism. In *Studies in Extended Metapsychology: Clinical Applications of Bion's Ideas*. London: Karnac.

Merleau-Ponty, Maurice. 1945, 1979. *Phenomenology of Perception*. Translated by Donald Landes. London: Routledge.

Meynen, Gerben. 2008. "Vrije Wil en Neurowetenschap." In *Kernproblemen van de Psychiatrie*, edited by J.A. den Boer, G. Glas, and A. Mooij, 25–42. Amsterdam: Boom.

Miller, Jacques-Alain. 1990. "Microscopia." In *Television: A Challenge to the Psychoanalytic Establishment*, edited by Jacques Lacan, xxxi–xxxv. New York-London: W.W. Norton & Company.

Monod, Jacques. 1970, 1971. *Chance and Necessity*. Translated by Austrin Wainhouse. New York: Alfred A. Knopf.

Mooij, Antoine. 2008. "Intentionaliteit en Causaliteit: De Inzet van de Fenomenologie." In *Kernproblemen van de Psychiatrie*, edited by J. A. den Boer, G. Glas, and A. Mooij, 195–212. Amsterdam: Boom.

Mooij, Antoine. 2010. "Intentionality and Causality: The Phenomenologic Case." In *Intentionality, Desire, Responsibility*, 1–22. Leiden-Boston: Brill Publishers.

Moyaert, Marianne. 2015. "From Religious Violence to Interreligious Hospitality." In *Paul Ricoeur in the Age of Hermeneutical Reason: Poetics, Praxis, and Critique*, edited by Roger Savage. Lanham, MA: Lexington Books.

Nagel, Thomas. 1974. "What Is It to Be a Bat?" *Philosophical Review* 83: 435–450.

Nagel, Thomas. 2001, 2016. *The Last Word*. Oxford: Oxford University Press.

Nietzsche, Friedrich. 1885, 1974. *Thus Spoke Zarathustra*. London: Penguin Books.

Nietzsche, Friedrich. 1887, 1998. *On the Genealogy of Morality: A Polemic*. Indianapolis: Hackett Publishing.

Nietzsche, Friedrich. 1895, 1976. The Antichrist. Trans. Walter Kaufmann. In *The Portable Nietzsche*. New York: Penguin.

Nietzsche, Friedrich. 1901, 2017. *The Will to Power*. London: Penguin Classics. Also on Internet: Gutenberg eBooks, Ebook-No. 52914.

Padel, Ruth. 1992. *Greek Images of the Tragic Self*. Princeton, NJ: Princeton University Press.

Parnas, Josef, Anna Urfer-Parnas, and Helle Stephensen. 2021. "Double Bookkeeping and Schizophrenia Spectrum: Divided Unified Phenomenal Consciousness." *European Archives of Psychiatry and Clinical Neuroscience* 271: 1513–1523.

Pfeijffer, Ilja Leonard. 2023. *Alkibiades*. Amsterdam-Antwerpen: Uitgeverij De Arbeiderspers.

Pilling, Stephen, Kate Clarke, Graham Parker, Katherine James, Stephen Landau, Tim Weaver, Roberta Razzagne, and Tom Craig. 2022. "Open Dialogue Compared to Treatment as Usual for Adults Experiencing Mental Health Crisis: Protocol for ODDESSI Multi-Site Cluster Randomised Controlled Trial." *Contemporary Clinical Trials* 113: 106664.

Pippin, Robert. 2018. *Hegel's Realm of Shadows: Logic as Metaphysics in Hegel's Science of Logic.* Chicago, IL: University of Chicago Press.

Plessner, Helmuth. 1975. *Die Stufen des Organischen und der Mensch.* Berlin/New York: De Gruyter.

Popper, Karl R., and John C. Eccles. 1977. *The Self and Its Brain: An Argument for Interactionism.* Berlin: Springer Verlag.

Postema, Johan. 2010. "Tot Hier... en Niet Verder." Accessed online: Wijsheden.com

Prigogine, Ilya, and Isabelle Stengers. 1985, 2018. *Order Out of Chaos.* New York: Verso Books.

Putnam, Hilary. 1981. "Brains in a Vat." In *Reason, Truth, and History*, 1–21. Cambridge: Cambridge University Press.

Rank, Otto. 1914, 2011. *The Double: A Psychoanalytic Study.* Chapel Hill: University of North Carolina Press.

Rey, Alain. 1995. *Le Robert: Dictionnaire Historique de la Langue Française.* Paris: Dictionnaires Le Robert.

Rohde, Erwin. 1893, 1925. *Psyche: Seelencult und Unsterblichkeitsglaube der Griechen.* Tübingen: Verlag von J.C.B. Mohr (Paul Siebeck).

Roudinesco, Élisabeth. 1986. *La Bataille de Cent Ans, Tome 1.* Paris: Éditions du Seuil.

Ruschmann, Erwin. 2013. "Transzendieren zur Transzendenz." *Zeitschrift für Spiritualität und Transzendentale Psychologie* 3 (2): 245–260.

Ryle, Gilbert. 1949, 1990. *The Concept of Mind.* London: Routledge.

Salvatore, Paola, Chittaranjan Bhuvaneswar, Mauricio Tohen, Hena-Maria Khalsa, Carlo Maggini, and Ross Baldessarini. 2014. "Capgras's Syndrome in First-Episode Psychotic Disorders." *Psychopathology* 47: 261–269.

Sartre, Jean-Paul. 1936, 1965. *La Transcendance de l'Ego: Esquisse d'une Description Phénoménologique.* Paris: Librairie Philosophique J. Vrin.

Sartre, Jean-Paul. 1940, 2010. *The Imaginary.* Germantown: Taylor & Francis Ltd.

Sartre, Jean-Paul. 1943. *L'Être et le Néant: Essai d'Ontologie Phénoménologique.* Paris: Éditions Gallimard.

Sartre, Jean-Paul. 1943, 2021. *Being and Nothingness.* Translated by Sarah Richmond. Washington, DC: Washington Square Press.

Sass, Louis A. 1994. *The Paradoxes of Delusion: Wittgenstein, Schreber, and the Schizophrenic Mind.* Ithaca and London: Cornell University Press.

Sass, Louis A., and Josef Parnas. 2003. "Schizophrenia, Consciousness, and the Self." *Schizophrenia Bulletin* 29 (3): 427–444.

Saussure, Ferdinand de. 1916, 1983. *Course in General Linguistics.* Translated by Roy Harris. Chicago, IL: Open Court Publishing Company.

Saussure, Ferdinand de. 2016. *Cours de Linguistique Générale.* Genève: Payot.

Scholte-Stalenhoeff, A. N., and R. J. van den Bosch. 2012. "Het Syndroom van Capgras: Convergerende Modellen." [Capgras' Syndrome: Converging Models.] *Tijdschrift voor Psychiatrie* 54 (12): 1011–1017.

Searle, John R. 1992. *The Rediscovery of the Mind.* Cambridge: MIT Press.

Seikkula, Jaakko. 2022. *Personal Announcement.*

Sérieux, Paul, and Jean Capgras. 1909, 1982. *Les Folies Raisonnantes: Le Délire d'Interprétation.* Marseille: Lafitte Reprints.

Smid, Dick, and Jim van Os. 2022. "De Praktijk Binnen de GGZ Is in Ontwikkeling, Volgt de Wetenschap?" [*The Practice within Mental Health Care Is Developing, Will Science Follow?*] *Tijdschrift voor Psychiatrie* 64: 87–93.

Solms, Mark. 2020. "Internet, YouTube Video," January 8, 2020.

Solms, Mark. 2021a. *De Verborgen Bron: Op Reis naar de Oorsprong van het Bewustzijn.* [*The Hidden Spring: A Revelatory New Theory of Consciousness That Returns Emotions to the Center of Mental Life.*] Amsterdam: Athenaeum-Polak & Van Gennep.

Solms, Mark. 2021b. *The Hidden Spring: A Journey to the Source of Consciousness.* New York-London: W. W. Norton & Company.

Spinoza, Benedict de. 1677, 2012. *Ethica.* Amsterdam: Boom.

Szasz, Thomas. 1961, 1974. *The Myth of Mental Illness: Foundations of a Theory of Personal Conduct.* New York: Harper and Row.

Vande Veire, Frank. 2015. *Tussen Blinde Fascinatie en Vrijheid: Het Mensbeeld bij Slavoj Žižek.* [*Between Blind Fascination and Freedom: The Image of Humanity in Slavoj Žižek.*] Nijmegen: Uitgeverij Vantilt.

Vanheule, Stijn. 2013. *Psychose anders bekeken: over het werk van Jacques Lacan.* [*Psychosis seen differently: on the work of Jacques Lacan.*] Leuven: LasnnooCampus.

Vanheule, Stijn. 2024. "Webimar Psychose", February 16, 2024.

Verhaeghe, Paul. 2001. "Mind Your Body: Lacan's Answer to a Classical Deadlock." In *Beyond Gender*, 20–36. New York: Other Press.

Vinkers, Dick J., Niek van der Lubbe, Ron de Reus, G. C. W. de Ruiter, and W. Pondaag. 2007. "Een 67-Jarige Vrouw Die Haar Dochter Voor een Dubbelganger Hield: De Differentiële Diagnostiek van Misidentificatie Wanen." *[A 67-Year-Old Woman Who Mistook Her Daughter for a Doppelganger: The Differential Diagnostics of Misidentification Delusions.] Nederlands Tijdschrift voor Geneeskunde* 151 (51): 2841–2844.

Wallon, Henri. 1949, 1983. *Les Origines du Caractère Chez l'Enfant.* Paris: Presses Universitaires de France, Quadrige.

Watsuji, Tetsurō. 1998. "The Japanese Spirit," "The Significance of Ethics as the Study of Man," and "The Way of the Japanese Subject." In *Sourcebook for Modern Japanese Philosophy: Selected Documents*, translated and edited by David Dilworth and Valdo Viglielmo, 231–287. Westport, CT: Greenwood Press.

Winnicott, Donald W. 1982. *The Maturational Processes and the Facilitating Environment.* London: The Hogarth Press.

Wolfson, Louis. 1970. *Le Schizo et les Langues.* Paris: Gallimard.

WVS. 2020. *Wet Verplichte GGZ en Wet Zorg en Dwang.* [Mandatory Mental Health Care Act.] The Hague: Ministerie van Volksgezondheid, Welzijn en Sport.

Žižek, Slavoy. 2006. *The Parallax View.* Cambridge MA: MIT Press.

Žižek, Slavoj. 2012. *Less than Nothing: Hegel and the Shadow of Dialectical Materialism.* New York: Verso Books.

INDEX OF NAMES

Achilles 8
Anderson, C.A. 59
Apuleius 83
Aristotles 118
Atta, K. 59

Badiou, A. 184
Bakhtin, M. xii, 137–140
Bally, C. 31n1
Barthes, R. 1, 23, 27, 161
Bateson, G. 1
Bergman, A. 33
Bergson, H. 66, 123–125, 127
Berrios, G.E. 60
Bhuvaneswar, C. 59
Bleuler, E. 16, 20–21
Blom, J.D. 49
Bonnefoi, C. 17
Bosch, R.J. van den 191
Brakel, L.A. 51

Capgras, J. 185, 191
Cassirer, E. 137
Chalmers, D.J. 13, 37, 76, 84–85, 92–93
Christodoulou, N. 59–60
Churchland, P. 13
Clérambault, G. de 51
Cohen, H. 137
Cotard, J. 49, 51

Damasio, A.R. 61, 182
Darby, R.R. 186
Darwin, C. 123
De Kesel, M. xii, 118–119, 178
Dennett, D. 8, 13
Dostoevsky, F.M. 186

Eccles, J. R. 191
Engel, G. 1, 7
Ettinger, B.L. 27
Evans, D. 89n3
Ey, H. 60

Filley, C.M. 59
Forlenza, N. 59
Foucault, M. 1–2, 14, 16–19, 21n2–21n3, 23, 27–28, 38, 66, 83, 92, 97, 120, 134, 141–143, 146, 150, 157, 161, 178
Fox, M.D. 186
Freud, S. xii, 8, 10n1, 13, 19–20, 24, 34, 49–50, 57n2, 60–62, 66, 75, 80, 89n3, 90, 103–105, 117–118, 139, 159–162, 175
Fromm, E. 187

Green, A. 44, 50
Gujski, M. 59

Haley, J. 1
Hashmi, S. 59
Hazif-Thomas, C. 51
Hegel, G.W.F. 15n1, 18, 103, 110, 113, 116, 121, 125–127, 150, 182

Heidegger, M. 24, 27, 32, 67, 71, 103, 108–117, 134, 150–151, 161, 167, 174, 179, 182–183
Heisenberg, W 25, 37–38, 75, 79
Hermes 10
Herter, H. 10
Hinshelwood, R.D. 95
Hoffmann, E.T.A. 188
Husserl, E. 15n1, 37, 66, 150, 167

Isaac, G. 59

Jackson, D.D. 1
Jackson, J.H. 60
Jaspers, K. 14, 15n1
Jonghe, F. de 60
Joseph, A.B. 60

Kalinova, M. 138
Kandel, E. 61, 85
Karskens, M. 19
Khalsa, H-M. 59
Kim, J. 37
Kopland, R. 9
Kraepelin, E. 188
Kristeva, J. 137, 174, 177
Kroon, J. de xiv–xv, 49, 66, 87–88, 104
Kusters, W. 81, 91
Kwant, R.C. 18

Lacan, J. xii–xiii, xv, 1–2, 9, 21n1, 23–29, 31n2, 32–35, 38, 40–41, 44–45, 49–50, 53–55, 57n1, 61–62, 66, 69, 71, 75–76, 80–81, 86–88, 89n3–89n4, 90–91, 93, 97–98, 109–111, 114, 116–125, 127, 129–130, 134–135, 138–140, 142–143, 145–148, 152, 156, 160–164, 168, 171, 174–175, 178, 181–182
Laganiere, S. 186
La mettrie, J. Offray de 6
Libet, B. 6
Lubbe, N. van der 192
Lütkehaus, L. 181

Maggini, C. 59
Mahler, M.S. 33
Margariti, M. 59
Markx, O. 60
Mauss, M. 190
Merleau-Ponty, M. 66, 68
Meynen, G. 6
Monod, J. 190
Muller, F. 83

Nagel, T. 8, 13, 85
Nietzsche, F. 17, 19, 103–105, 105n1, 108–114, 116, 150, 182

Padel, R. 190
Pascual-Leone, A. 186
Pine, F. 33
Pondaag, W. 192
Popper, K.R. 191
Prasad, S. 186
Prigogine, I. 51
Putnam, H. 8, 13

Raboul-Lachaaux 185
Reus, R. de 192
Rey, A. 83
Rohde, E. 10
Roudinesco, E. 191
Ruiter, G.C.W. de 192

Salvatore, P. 59
Sartre, J-P. 13, 67, 71, 75, 81, 91, 110–111, 113–116, 138, 167, 179
Saussure, F. de 2, 15, 23–24, 26–29, 87, 97, 133, 137, 143, 161
Scholte-Stalenhoeff, A.N. 191
Schopenhauer, A. 67, 181
Searle, J.R. 7–8, 76, 84–85
Sechehaye, A. 31n1
Seikkula, J. xii–xiii, 1, 138–139
Sérieux, P. 191
Solms, M. 5, 38, 85, 161
Stengers, I. 51
Szasz, T. 16, 20

Todorov, T. 137
Tohen, M. 59

Vande Veire, F. 122
Veen, P.H.F. van 83
Verhaeghe, P. 192
Verplancke, T. 49, 66, 88
Vinkers, D.J. 192

Weakland, J.H. 1

Zeno van Elea 8, 66–67
Žižek, S. 1, 79, 121–127, 134–135, 182–183

INDEX OF SUBJECTS

alienation 24, 35, 48, 53, 55, 61–62, 72, 113, 128, 135, 148, 155, 162, 182
automatisme mental 51

black hole 17, 36–37, 69, 91, 133
black matter 36–37

castration 24, 28, 31n2, 32, 35, 41, 50, 81, 86, 88, 91, 161
connotation 20, 25, 77, 97, 107
contingency 29, 109, 111, 113, 126

delusion 9, 14, 25, 42, 44, 47, 51, 53, 55–56, 76, 81–82, 90–92, 95–96, 98, 148, 181
Delusional Misidentification Syndrome (DMS) 59
denotation 77, 97
desire 5, 8, 17, 20, 24–26, 32, 34, 38–39, 41, 75–76, 78, 80–81, 84, 86, 88, 89n3, 90–91, 93, 104, 109–111, 114, 116, 119–121, 123–125, 127–128, 132, 134–135, 137, 146–149, 152–157, 159, 161–164, 170–177, 181–183
determinism 13, 36
dialectics 29, 39, 79, 81, 91, 110, 113, 125, 127, 140, 175, 182
doppelganger 9, 35, 58–59, 61–62, 69, 88, 92
doubling 62, 69
DSM-5 (*Diagnostic and Statistical Manual*) 7, 70, 85
dualism 8, 13, 40, 84, 150

ecology of mind 1
empirism, empirical 15n1, 68, 93, 95, 118, 122, 125, 153–154, 156, 166–167, 171
exotopy 188
exteriority 34–35, 138, 148
extime, extimity 109

fause route 2
foreclosure of the Name-of-the-Father 44, 53, 145
freedom 3, 6, 13, 17–18, 25, 28, 30, 39–41, 77, 81–82, 91–92, 97, 111, 113, 115, 167, 170, 172, 176, 179

gap 5, 14, 16, 24–26, 32, 34–42, 45, 53–54, 58, 65, 67–71, 77, 95, 97, 110–111, 114, 119–120, 123–128, 135, 139, 147
grammar 28
graph, complicated 69, 96, 142
graph, simple 10, 53, 77, 93, 130, 142

hallucination 14, 25, 42, 44, 50–51, 53, 66, 68, 70, 76, 81, 89n3, 90–91, 95–96, 148, 181

identity 9, 14, 24, 26–27, 29–30, 31n2, 34–35, 44, 47, 49, 53–55, 66, 69–72, 75, 79, 86–87, 111, 114, 119, 128–129, 131, 133–134, 136, 138–140, 143–145, 148, 152–154, 156, 169, 174–175
imaginary 9, 32, 34–35, 39–40, 42, 44–45, 47–56, 58, 61–62, 69–70, 72–73, 75, 80–81, 86, 90–91, 111, 117, 122, 129–131, 144–145, 148, 161
intimacy 48
intuism xiv, 3, 7, 96, 122, 152

language 7, 10–11, 14, 19, 21n4, 23–30, 33, 36–37, 39–40, 44, 48, 52–56, 57n1, 65, 67, 69–70, 72, 75–78, 80, 82–84, 86–88, 91–93, 97–99, 105, 108–110, 117–121, 123–124, 127–131, 134, 136–139, 143–148, 151–153, 156–157, 161–165, 167–172, 174–182

Marburg, school van 137
market forces 12
materialism 13, 38, 93, 125–127, 132, 183
matter 8–10, 18–19, 36, 39–40, 58, 77–78, 85, 101, 105, 107, 110, 112, 121, 125–126, 178
mechanistic model 99
mirror stage 24, 32–35, 53, 61–62, 75, 81, 83, 86, 91, 161
monism 13, 32, 92, 132

narcissism 34, 50, 61–62
negative hallucination 5, 9, 14, 43–44, 49–52, 65–71, 81–82, 86, 91–92
negative matter 36–37
neuropsychoanalysis 5, 38, 161
nihilistic delusion 47, 49–56, 76, 81–82, 91–92
nomenclature 29
nothing, nothingness 5, 8–10, 12, 23–26, 32, 35–45, 47, 50, 52–54, 56, 58, 64–73, 75–76, 79–82, 89n3, 90–92, 101, 103–125, 127–128, 130–131, 133–134, 143, 157, 159, 161, 163–165, 167–168, 170–183
nucleus amygdala 157

objectivism, objectivity 25–26, 37–38, 41, 75, 78–79, 97, 141, 144, 149, 153–157, 164, 166, 171, 175
open dialogue xii–xiii, 1, 132, 139, 141, 168–169
outsidedness 137–139

paradigm shift 40, 54
paradox 8, 18, 66–67, 112–115, 129–131, 162
paranoidism 60, 88, 95–96
parole 19, 21n4, 23, 28–29
phenomenology 11, 15, 15n1, 19, 42n1, 68, 71, 152, 154, 167, 169
physicalization, physicalistic 6–7, 13–14, 18, 29, 40, 82, 166, 169
proprioception, propriocepsis 35
psychiatry xii, 1–3, 5–21, 25–26, 29–30, 36, 38, 40, 47–49, 51–52, 54, 56, 59–60, 63, 66, 68, 70–71, 75–79, 81, 84–85, 89n1, 90–99, 101, 122, 132–137, 141–146, 148–150, 152–157, 166–173, 175–177, 181
psychology 5–7, 11, 19–20, 24–26, 28–30, 38, 76, 85, 92, 118
psychosis 1–2, 9, 12, 25, 41–42, 44, 49, 52–56, 58, 60–63, 65–66, 72–73, 76–78, 82–83, 85, 90, 92, 94–98, 117, 121, 134, 137, 142–145, 148, 150, 152, 162, 165, 168, 178, 180–181, 183

rapprochement (fase) 33
reductionism 12, 37, 59, 77, 84–85, 98, 136, 144–145, 151, 166
rhizome 142

schizophrenia 18, 21, 60, 122, 167–168
science 5, 7, 10, 13–14, 16, 19, 23, 25, 28–30, 35–38, 40–41, 48, 51, 69, 75, 78–89, 103–105, 109–116, 119–120, 141–142, 146, 153, 161, 166, 173, 179–181
scission see castration
scotomisation 53, 66
separation 5, 9, 24, 27–29, 31n2, 32, 35–36, 41–42, 50, 58, 67, 71–72, 75–76, 81, 86–88, 90–91, 93, 128, 146, 161–164, 174, 176, 182

sign 7, 23–24, 27, 29, 35–36, 38, 41, 49, 87, 106–107, 119, 124, 136, 143, 164
signified (*signifié*) 23–24, 27, 29, 87, 120, 124, 143
signifier (*significant*) 11–12, 14, 16, 23–25, 27–29, 47–48, 55–56, 60, 64, 66, 79, 83–85, 87–88, 92, 117, 120–121, 123–124, 129–131, 139, 143, 147, 150, 153–154, 161, 163, 169
structuralism xiv, 8–9, 15–16, 18, 23–31, 75, 77, 79, 92, 97–99, 132, 135, 137–139, 143–144, 149, 152, 161
structure 2, 9, 18, 21n4, 24–30, 39, 54–55, 60–61, 70–72, 76–77, 86–87, 93, 96, 98, 103–104, 118, 120, 132–137, 139, 142–146, 148, 151–152, 159–161, 164–165, 167–168, 174, 178–179
subject, subjective xv, 1–2, 5–6, 8–10, 13–14, 16, 19, 21n1, 24–27, 29, 31n2, 32–42, 42n1, 48–56, 64, 68, 70–72, 75–89, 89n3, 97–99, 105, 117–123, 127, 132–133, 138–139, 141–153, 156, 162–164, 166–169, 171–183
symbolic 9, 14, 21n1, 24–26, 29–30, 31n2, 32, 34–35, 38–42, 44, 47–49, 51–56, 57n1, 58, 61–64, 67, 69–73, 75–77, 79, 81–82, 84, 86–88, 89n3, 90–91, 93, 97–98, 110–111, 117, 120, 122, 124–125, 127, 129–131, 133–139, 142–149, 151–152, 154–156, 161–172, 174–181
symbolization 29, 33, 35, 40, 42, 49, 53–54, 61, 63, 67, 70–71, 80–81, 86–87, 91, 110, 123–124, 162–163, 165, 174, 177
syndrome (Cotard's/Capgras') 5, 9, 35, 43–44, 47–63, 66, 69, 88
syntaxis 28

transcendence, transcendent 5, 10, 13, 24, 27, 37, 40, 80, 90, 116, 122, 125–127, 151–152, 157, 161, 166–173, 176–177, 182–183

uncertainty factor 26, 30, 38, 69, 77, 98–99, 113, 116, 127, 170, 172, 177
unconscious 15–16, 24–26, 38, 50, 65, 68, 84, 88, 98, 104, 118, 120, 139, 146, 159, 162–163, 175, 181
United Kingdom 137
United States 137

[illegible]